Patient Citizens, Immigrant Mothers

Critical Issues in Health and Medicine

Edited by Rima D. Apple, University of Wisconsin–Madison,
and Janet Golden, Rutgers University, Camden

Growing criticism of the U.S. health care system is coming from consumers, politicians, the media, activists, and health care professionals. Critical Issues in Health and Medicine is a collection of books that explores these contemporary dilemmas from a variety of perspectives, among them political, legal, historical, sociological, and comparative, and with attention to crucial dimensions such as race, gender, ethnicity, sexuality, and culture.

For a list of titles in the series, see the last page of the book.

Patient Citizens, Immigrant Mothers

Mexican Women, Public Prenatal Care, and the Birth-Weight Paradox

Alyshia Gálvez

Rutgers University Press

New Brunswick, New Jersey, and London

Library of Congress Cataloging-in-Publication Data

Gálvez, Alyshia.
  Patient citizens, immigrant mothers : Mexican women, public prenatal care, and the birth-weight paradox / Alyshia Gálvez.
    p. cm. — (Critical issues in health and medicine)
  Includes bibliographical references and index.
  ISBN 978–0–8135–5141–8 (hardcover : alk. paper) — ISBN 978–0–8135–5142–5 (pbk. : alk. paper)
    1. Women—Mexico—Social conditions.   2. Women immigrants—United States—Social conditions.   3. Prenatal care—United States.   4. Childbirth—United States—Cross-cultural studies.   I. Title.
  HQ1462.G35   2011
  306.874′30896872073—dc22

                                                                                        2011001050

A British Cataloging-in-Publication record for this book is available from the British Library.

Visit our Web site: http://rutgerspress.rutgers.edu

Manufactured in the United States of America

For Lázaro, Elías, and Carlos, always

Contents

Acknowledgments

This book has benefited by the generous input and support of a number of colleagues and institutions. Of course, the errors that inevitably remain in the text are mine alone. I had the opportunity to present grant proposals, the research plan, and drafts of the manuscript in various settings. These opportunities steered me away from many errors in direction and approach and also gave me encouragement along the way.

Funding for the research described here was provided by PSC-CUNY faculty grants and New York University's University Research Challenge Fund. In addition, a teaching fellowship in New York University's Center for Latin American and Caribbean Studies from 2005 to 2007 as well as a semester leave from Lehman College in 2009 gave me the time, space, and resources I needed to conduct research and write. I am grateful to the institutions that made the research possible by offering institutional review or access to research sites or both: Asociación Tepeyac de New York, City University of New York, Lehman College of the City University of New York, Manhattan Hospital Center (a pseudonym), New York University School of Medicine, and New York University Graduate School of Arts and Sciences.

Working groups and informal groupings of colleagues at the following institutions read chapters, listened to me talk about my study formally and informally, and with their comments and suggestions deeply enriched the project. I extend thanks to the members of Body, Belief, and Bioethics, a working group chaired in 2005–2006 by Rayna Rapp and Faye Ginsburg of the Center for Religion and Media, New York University; my cohort at the 2010 CUNY Faculty Fellowship Publication Program; and the faculty of Sociomedical Sciences at the Mailman School of Public Health at Columbia University. Talks at Brown, Rutgers, Syracuse, and Fordham universities, the Graduate Center of CUNY, and the Universidad Iberoamericana de Puebla brought this and my former research program together.

Many individuals contributed to this work in large and small ways. First and foremost, I am grateful to the many women who sat with me and shared their lives even while their children became bored and their babies fussed. Although I sometimes won a smile from little ones with markers, snacks, and games, this was poor compensation for stealing their mothers' attention. The generosity of the women and their families who participated in this study, even while I offered them little in return, was moving and humbling. I am thankful for the kind assistance of the following people who gave me access to field sites, endured my annoying queries and requests, and offered sound guidance on the formulation of my research questions: María Zúñiga Barba, Eric Manheimer, Machelle Allen, the medical and ancillary staff at the hospital, Valeriana and Patricia Pizarro, Kristen Norget, Teresa García, Megan Martin, Rosa María Tellez, and Khiara Bridges. Valeriana holds a special place in our family's hearts for her healing work with our son while we were in Oaxaca. Manuela Fuentes, Saúl Pacheco, their children and families in New York and in the state of Puebla, including Moisés Fuentes, have been exceedingly generous and welcoming for years and my family deeply values their friendship: *mil gracias por la amistad y convivencia, los queremos*. A special thanks to Monserrat Xilotl, who gave so generously of her time and was incredibly helpful—having the Mexican consul's wife as a research assistant and valuable interlocutor was a privilege I never expected and for which I am grateful.

Thanks are due to Marlie Wasserman, Peter Guarnaccia, and Pamela Fischer for their enthusiasm about and commitment to the project at Rutgers University Press, and to my editor there, Peter Mickulas, for his professionalism, humor, and patience.

Although we may presume teaching is for the benefit of students, I have always found quite the opposite: that I learn far more from my students than I could ever offer to them. To the students who helped with this project, primary thanks are due to Sandra Céspedes, whose expert transcriptions and formatting assistance were key, and to Elizabeth Capone-Henríquez, who did tremendous work on the bibliography and statistical sleuthing in the project's early phases. Karen Rojas Chávez did important formatting work at the end of this project. Others who started out as students but have become friends and colleagues and to whom I am grateful include Catarina Reiland, Eva Blom Raison, Maya Vaughan-Smith, Miguel Angeles, Melissa Maldonado-Salcedo, and Laura Rivera. The following Lehman College colleagues made helpful interventions into my own political economy of scholarly production and also contributed to an atmosphere of collegiality at key junctures: Laird Bergad, Ricardo Fernández, Licia Fiol-Matta, Timothy Alborn, Milagros Ricourt, David Badillo, Luisa Borrell, Victoria Sanford, Marlene Gottlieb, Marie Marianetti, Bertrade Banoum, and Susan Markens. Colleagues and mentors at other institutions also offered or participated in key opportunities to share and discuss the research publicly and privately: Faye Ginsburg, Rayna Rapp, Jennifer Hirsch, Suzanne Oboler, Anahí Viladrich, Aminata Maraesa, Diana Taylor, Margarita Alegría, Elise Andaya, Leigh Binford, Nina Siulc, Sherine Hamdy, Marge Lunney,

Alice Lun, Eleanor Kehoe, Soyeon Cho, Matthew Gutmann, Marcela Ibarra Mateos, Joanne Csete, Peter Messeri, Virginia Rauh, Glenn Hendler, William Kelleher, Natasha Iksander, Alexandra Délano, Lina Newton, Ramona Hernández, Elena Sabogal, Victoria Hattam, Judith Hellman, Leslie Martino, Becca Howes-Mischel, Leticia Calderón-Chelius, Juan Martínez Louvier, Lesley Sharp, and Renato Rosaldo. Sari Lapin-Mayer and Andrea Maldonado very generously proofread the manuscript, saving me from many embarrassing errors.

I would like to thank the friends and their families who support me and my work always: Alex Atkin, Alicia Carmona, Kelly Collins, Denis Pareja, Louisa Plous, Alison and Jessica Ritz and their dad, David, Jenny Steingart, Robert O'Hagan, Jamie Berk and Andrew Walker, Sandro and Gya CereShin, Gastón and Marisol Arancibia, Cybele Lyle, Stacy Tolchin, Angie Armer, Leah Mundell, Jessie Temple, and Marika Lynch. And thanks also to my family: Kathy and Eric Blond, Daniel Blond, Sarafina and Patricia Rom, Darcy and Darrin Bishop, Heidi Keller, Rosemary and Gene Matrejek, Blanca García, Sergio Rodríguez and family, Elizabeth Gálvez and family, and Elizabeth Buckner. My grandmother, Margaret Buckner, very nearly made it to the century mark; if she had, she would have seen and been especially happy about this book. Finally, a special thank you and all my love to my favorite people: Lázaro, Elías, and Carlos Gálvez.

Patient Citizens, Immigrant Mothers

Chapter 1

Paradoxes and Patients

Immigrants and Prenatal Care

When Marisol (a pseudonym) was pregnant with her first child in her home-town, a rural hamlet outside the state capital of Puebla, Mexico, she suffered frequently from morning sickness. Her mother-in-law, with whom she and her husband lived, knew a solution. When the nausea was too much for her daughter-in-law to bear, she would prepare *caldo de gallina*, chicken soup. She wrung an older, egg-laying hen's neck, plucked it, and over several hours cooked a rich broth laden with vegetables picked from the fields surrounding their home.[1] When Marisol sipped the soup, served with fresh, hand-made corn tortillas, her nausea subsided. During her second pregnancy, having migrated to New York City with her husband and child, Marisol again suffered from morning sickness. Because her mother-in-law's soup could not bridge the dis-tance, Marisol asked her obstetrician at her monthly visit to a public prenatal clinic what she should do. He responded that she should buy a box of crackers and keep it handy, eating a few before getting out of bed and whenever she felt queasy. I asked her what she thought of that advice. She replied, "It's so practi-cal! The box of crackers costs a dollar. I can find them at any corner store, and I can keep them next to my bed or in my purse when I'm out of the house. It's much easier than cooking soup all day!"

This vignette illustrates how one woman cared for herself and the ways the advice and care she was given by others differed between two pregnancies. Marisol does not say that the chicken soup was not effective for combating nau-sea; she was clear that it was. However, for her second pregnancy, she shifted her practices (and, by extension, her nutritional intake) to adapt to the advice she was given by a physician, whom she described as being more knowledgeable than her mother-in-law. She also adapted to a changed set of circumstances in which crackers—convenient, inexpensive, and easily accessible—seemed preferable and more suited to her new life in New York City. Meanwhile, her physician never asked her how she combated nausea in her previous pregnancy. Had she been asked, she might have mentioned the caldo de gallina, and it is possible her provider might have suggested she try chicken soup again rather than recommend a nutritionally inferior, processed food.

This book is based on an ethnographic study that sought answers to the following questions: How are conflicting approaches to pregnancy care reconciled by Mexican immigrant women? How do they decide which aspects of self-care to adopt and which to reject? What impact do the attitudes of prenatal care providers in public clinics toward immigrant patients have on their experiences of pregnancy and childbirth and on the outcomes?

The Birth-Weight Paradox

In 2003, at a conference on Mexican immigration to New York City at City College, a Columbia Presbyterian Medical Center surgeon, Carlos Navarro, said, "Mexican immigrant women have healthy babies. They have some sort of cultural advantage, but we [doctors] don't know what it is." With this statement, Navarro implicitly issued a powerful call for ethnography. Historically, that which is "cultural," as opposed to that which is psychological or biological, has been the terrain of inquiry for cultural anthropologists and the object of their preferred methodology, ethnography. This methodology opts for an inductive approach that seeks to solve research questions by examining the everyday experiences, discourses, and practices of individuals and groups. Anthropologist Aihwa Ong argues for ethnography: "As anthropologists, we are skeptical of grand theories. We pose big questions through the prism of situated ethnographic research on disparate situations of contemporary living" (2006, 12).

This book examines the purported cultural advantage of Mexican immigrant women in pregnancy and childbirth and the puzzle identified by epidemiologists as the "birth-weight paradox." This is a subset of the "immigrant paradox," in which first-generation immigrants have more favorable health indicators, by some measures, than their U.S.-born counterparts (Forbes and Frisbie 1991; Landale, Oropesa, and Gorman 1999; Rumbaut and Weeks 1996), and of the "Latino health paradox," in which Latinos demonstrate an advantage over other groups on a number of health indicators (Alegría et al. 2008; Escobar and Vega 2006; Fuller et al. 2009; Taningco 2007; Vega, Rodríguez, and Gruskin 2009).

The birth-weight paradox, also sometimes called the Latina paradox, is that immigrant women born in some Latin American countries with a high prevalence of "risk factors" nevertheless have a "perinatal advantage": they have fewer low-birth-weight infants than other groups. Mothers born in Mexico, among a few other immigrant-sending countries, tend to have lower rates of pregnancy complications, such as low birth weight, premature births, intrauterine growth retardation, and infant mortality, than might be predicted by their "disadvantageous risk profiles" (Morenoff 2000, 12; also Buekens et al. 2000; Cramer 1987; Forbes and Frisbie 1991; Hessol and Fuentes-Afflick 2000; Landale, Oropesa, and Gorman 2000; Liu and Laraque 2006; Palloni and Morenoff 2001; Taningco 2007). Low birth weight is a useful measure of birth outcomes because it is an indication of infants born "too small," "too soon," or both. It is an important indicator of risk for neonatal mortality, but even more broadly it is "an important predictor of a number of health and developmental outcomes" (Conley, Strully, and Bennet 2003, 10). This rupture in the formula that "wealth equals health" is considered paradoxical because it conflicts with expectations that poorer women with greater "risk" factors will have more complicated pregnancies and childbirths and because this protection declines over time—greater assimilation into the U.S. health care system results in worse outcomes (Hayes-Bautista 2002; also Alegría et al. 2007; Cook et al. 2009).

Hypotheses for the birth-weight paradox, some of which apply to the broader Latino health paradox, include the "salmon-bias," "healthy-migrant," dietary, "health-behaviors," and acculturation hypotheses. The salmon-bias hypothesis is premised on the idea that immigrants return to their communities of origin on retirement or illness, thus becoming "statistically immortal" (Abraído-Lanza et al. 1999; Palloni and Arias 2004). The healthy-migrant hypothesis holds that those who migrate tend to be healthier in the first place than those they leave behind and healthier than the native-born population as a whole (Abraído-Lanza et al. 1999; Shai and Rosenwaike 1987; Sorlie et al. 1993). Dietary hypotheses hold that Mexican immigrants eat more protein and consume more vitamins and minerals than their native-born counterparts and that such a diet contributes to favorable birth outcomes (Guendelman and Abrams 1995). The health-behaviors hypothesis suggests that Latinos practice more favorable health behaviors and have fewer risk factors than non-Latinos. According to the acculturation hypothesis, as the length of time immigrants reside in the United States increases, a rise in unhealthy behaviors like smoking and alcohol intake is likely, as is a higher body mass index (Abraído-Lanza, Chao, and Flórez 2005). This hypothesis predicts that cultures of origin offer protective features, such as positive attitudes about pregnancy, and that these factors favor good birth outcomes and are eroded as immigrants become increasingly acculturated (Landale, Oropesa, and Gorman 1999; Rumbaut and Weeks 1996; Santiago-Irizarry 1996; Scribner and Dwyer 1989; see also Alegría et al. 2007; Hunt, Schneider, and Comer 2004; Mulvaney-Day, Alegría, and Sribney 2007; Singh and Siahpush 2001). Even so, scholars have cautioned that studies of acculturation are insufficiently multidimensional and fail to take sufficient account of structural as well as cultural factors (Abraído-Lanza et al. 2006). None of these hypotheses has been conclusively proven, leaving the paradox to be described as an elusive mystery (Abraído-Lanza 1999; Frank and Hummer 2002; Harley 2004) or dismissed as the product of statistical error, bias, and an insistence on expecting poor outcomes from minority social actors (Palloni and Arias 2004; Palloni and Morenoff 2001; Santiago-Irizarry 1996; Wilson 2008).

The risk factors associated with low birth weight and infant death cited in studies of the birth-weight paradox include socioeconomic and behavioral correlates of expectant women such as low income, low levels of education, late or no prenatal care, being a teen mother or of advanced maternal age, being an unmarried mother, parity (or birth order, first-borns are at greater risk), insufficient spacing between births, lack of access to health insurance, alcohol consumption, smoking and drug abuse, and being employed, as well as physical factors like slight maternal stature, inadequate maternal weight gain, and low maternal weight before pregnancy (Conley, Strully, and Bennet 2003, 12). These risk factors are exceedingly problematical, as will be discussed further, but they are the ones that are operational in many epidemiological approaches to birth outcomes. Although more strictly medical causes, such as maternal infection or other health problems, placental problems, and birth defects, are associated with low birth weight and infant death, they are not considered elements of the birth-weight paradox. Moreover, protective factors have been hypothesized to contribute to the favorable birth outcomes of Latina women, including cultural factors like a good diet, social support, religious faith, and positive attitudes regarding pregnancy (Fernández and Newby 2010; Viruell-Fuentes 2006; Guendelman and Abrams 1995; Harley 2004; Scribner 1996; Scribner and Dwyer 1989; Sherraden and Barrera 1996; Viruell-Fuentes and Schulz 2009; see also Mulvaney-Day, Alegría, and Sribney 2007).

The paradox is evident in New York City, the primary location of this study, where Mexican immigrant women have relatively low rates of infant mortality and low birth weight in spite of higher incidences of many "risk" factors (New York City Department of Health and Mental Hygiene 2008). From 2002 to 2008, the mortality rate for infants of women born in Mexico was 4.32 per 1000 births as opposed to 5.91 for the city as a whole. Only 5.8 percent of

Mexican mothers gave birth to a low-birth-weight infant (under 2500 grams), versus 8.8 percent for the city as a whole for the same years. These outcomes occurred in spite of the fact that the Mexican mothers had a uniformly unfavorable number of the major risk factors associated with low birth weight and infant mortality. Of the factors that were tracked in the New York City *Summary of Vital Statistics* for these years, Mexican mothers were more likely to be unmarried, on Medicaid, a teenager, and to have late or no prenatal care (Begier et al. 2010).[2] Although the New York City public-hospital system and health department have invested a great deal of effort and resources in campaigns to decrease the rates of infant mortality and low birth weight, the rates for Mexican immigrant women have remained steadily low since the turn of the century.[3]

Another aspect of the birth-weight paradox is its limited duration. The perinatal advantage is most pronounced for Latina women who have themselves migrated (first generation). The comparative advantage declines over time and across generations, as immigrants and their children become increasingly socialized and adapted to life in the United States (Alegría et al. 2007; Guendelman and Abrams 1995; Hunt, Schneider, and Comer 2004; Landale, Oropesa, and Gorman 1999; Mulvaney-Day, Alegría, and Sribney 2007; Rumbaut and Weeks 1996; Santiago-Irizarry 1996; Scribner and Dwyer 1989; Singh and Siahpush 2001). For the second and further generations, birth outcomes come progressively to resemble those of others who share similar socioeconomic status (Cook et al. 2009). In essence, the more recent a woman's migration, the more likely her wealth does not predict her health; with longer stays in the United States, socioeconomic status becomes a more reliable predictor of health outcomes than ethnicity is. In New York City, births to Mexican mothers are still overwhelmingly to women who are first-generation immigrants. Nonetheless, it is possible to discern the beginning of a shift characterized by the growth of a second generation (women of Mexican ancestry born in the United States), increased consumption of prenatal care, and use of the Medicaid system. Even so, rates of infant mortality and low birth weight have stayed about the same. Although intuitively one might assume that increased participation in the public health system would improve outcomes, data gathered in other locations with longer-standing Mexican immigrant communities and deep generational sedimentation indicate that we can expect to see a decline in the birth outcomes of Mexican mothers in New York City in the coming years (Landale, Oropesa, and Gorman 1999; Rumbaut and Weeks 1996). At a conference, Marcelo Suárez-Orozco (2009), co-director of the interdisciplinary institute Immigration Studies @ NYU, quipped that immigrant visas to the

United States should be stamped with a warning: the United States is a "danger to your health" (also Alegría et al. 2007; Santora 2006; *Unnatural Causes* 2007; Vega and Amaro 1994).

Early studies of the health paradox did not differentiate based on nativity status (Williams, Binkin, and Clingman 1986), nationality, or immigration history at all, lumping Hispanics indiscriminately (Forbes and Frisbie 1991). Later studies, though, have examined the birth-weight paradox over time and across populations. Some studies (Abraído-Lanza et al. 1999; Guendelman and Abrams 1995; Scribner and Dwyer 1989) have compared the birth outcomes of women who were born in Mexico with women who are the daughters or grand-daughters of Mexican immigrants, the second and third generations following migration.

This book looks at two interrelated phenomena associated with the birth-weight paradox: first, the practices engaged in by Mexican immigrants to care for their pregnancies and, second, the decline of those practices, which it becomes clear is not a slow erosion but a rapid shedding that can be expected to have deleterious effects over time. This study examines women's experiences during pregnancy and childbirth both before and after migration and the ways they negotiate the advice and care they receive in public prenatal clinics.

Sociomedical sciences and qualitative public health research seek to identify the social determinants of health and to trace the biological pathways of social status, inequality, and behaviors.[4] This study, and all similarly qualitative, ethnographic research, is challenged by the difficulty, if not impossibility, of demonstrating a correlation between behaviors and health outcomes (see Conley, Strully, and Bennet 2003, 55). Although quantitative and longitudinal research will always be necessary to show long-term trends and the impact of public health interventions, qualitative studies such as this can suggest ways to orient such research.

Many studies have looked at these phenomena in other regions in the United States, but none, to date, has interpreted Mexican immigrant women's pregnancy and childbirth experiences in the context of their immigration stories. I contend that women's status as immigrants has explanatory force both for the healthful and protective practices they bring to their pregnancies and also for the eagerness with which they embrace dominant biomedical models of care. It explains the rapidity in the decline of some cultural practices faster than would occur with the erosion of memory or the gap of generations. It gives us a way to account for the participation of women in giving up practices with which they were raised even while the efficacy of such practices is still evident.

The Pace and Causes of Change in Pregnancy Care

This study indicates that an erosion of the protective benefits that Mexican women bring to their lives in the United States may occur even within the course of individual women's reproductive histories. Marisol's story about chicken soup illustrates changes in one woman's diet preceding and following migration to the United States; it reveals how the pregnancy-related practices and habits of women can shift. By examining how individual women alter the ways they care for their pregnancies over the course of their reproductive lives and immigration experiences, we can see how women reconcile ideas about pregnancy and childbirth that they gathered in their hometowns and from their mothers and grandmothers with new information obtained in New York City.

The processes by which women cease to engage in the self-care practices that are familiar to them from their communities in which they grew up are complex. They do not unquestioningly embrace the models of care they perceive to be dominant in New York. Women weigh the benefits and costs of different models of care, critique the faults they see in each, and strive to do what they perceive is best for themselves and their children given their current knowledge and resources. At the same time, they are funneled into a system in which their status as "Medicaid patients," immigrants, and often bearers of multiple "risk factors" is a means to categorize them and indoctrinate them into norms of behavior expected in the public health context of New York City and, by extension, in the larger sphere of public benefits. All these processes occur in the context of immigration, which is not merely circumstantial but an absolutely central aspect of their management of the information, habits, and expertise they bring with them and those they encounter here. They are often enthusiastic that they are able to access a well-equipped, hospital-based prenatal clinic and are inclined to view the advice given them in such settings as inherently superior to the care surrounding pregnancy and birth in their communities of origin.

Further, women describe the prestige associated with accessing the means to perform certain modern identities, such as having a baby in a hospital, as a privilege associated with migration. Jennifer Hirsch notes that, "in common usage, the word modern implies a contrast with the traditional, a description of the way things are now in comparison to how they have been in the past" (2003, 13). When describing their marriages, the participants in her study said that, compared with their parents' relationships, their own were "*better*— supposedly freer from constraint, more pleasurable and satisfying, perhaps even in some way more prestigious. The prestige of modernity is so omnipresent a feature of our intellectual landscape as to be invisible; it has become one of our unexamined habits of thought" (13).

Hirsch and her colleagues write, "Gender is deployed as a trope to represent progress or its lack. . . . Men and women . . . use gendered idioms to express their yearning for modernity or their melancholy at the waning of tradition" (2010, 9). In a similar vein, in her research in Cameroon, Jennifer Johnson-Hanks traced the choices of Beti women regarding contraception as a mode for the expression of modern gendered identities, as a way to pursue a "disciplined, honorable and modern identity" (2002, 231–232). Contraception choice offers a mode of "'self-actualization' . . . [historically denied Beti women but available to them in] sexual and marital relationships and childbearing: managing the timing and social context of sex, marriage, and especially motherhood" (233). These uses of the concept of modernity are similar to the efforts of women in the present study to manage their pregnancies as well as child-rearing within conceptualizations of modern, migrant identities. The prestige of biomedicine is not limited to women's tenure in the United States but is a feature of life in rural Mexico as well as in the globalized, transnational spaces of migration.

Nonetheless, the efforts of families to access such tokens of prestige as biomedical care have hazards. It will become clear in later chapters that the changes and compromises Mexican immigrant women make toward achieving their aspirations may have unintended consequences and long-term repercussions in the realm of health, as well as in the supraindividual realm of immigrant integration.

Change and progress are not the same thing. As Hirsch succinctly puts it, "Modernity is a cultural construction and a product of social transformations that has both costs and benefits" (2003, 14). This conclusion is similar to those drawn by anthropologists Valentina Napolitano in her work on vernacular modernities (2002) and Matthew Gutmann in his on modern gendered identities (1996), both in Mexico. Cultural changes made in the name of modernity can reinforce inequalities or create new ones, can push out sound traditional practices and their practitioners as relics. These processes can also contribute to neoliberal subject formations in which the state is absolved of responsibility for its citizen and noncitizen members, and self-formation becomes an act of citizenship. Ong describes this phenomenon as follows: "Neoliberal policies of 'shrinking' the state are accompanied by a proliferation of techniques to remake the social and citizen-subjects. Thus neoliberal logic requires populations to be free, self-managing, and self-enterprising individuals in different spheres of everyday life—health, education, [and] bureaucracy" (2006, 14). Rebecca

Howes-Mischel (forthcoming), Andrea Maldonado (2010b), and Vania Smith-Oka (forthcoming) similarly trace the promotion of a neoliberal model of citizenship in contemporary Mexico and the withdrawal of the state from providing services in favor of a model emphasizing "self-care." Later, I will describe the intersection of state-generated notions of self-care with the web of practices women describe having learned from their female kin in their hometowns.

A growing emphasis on self-care in Mexico is particularly relevant to the postures and attitudes of Mexican immigrants in the United States. Self-care can be taken to extremes: for lack of viable options in their hometowns, migrant families take it upon themselves to migrate to a new country where they hope to achieve access to the resources they associate with economic stability, upward mobility, health, and well-being. Indeed, in an exchange that illustrates the honor and pitfalls of such processes, Mexican President Vicente Fox (2000–2006) repeatedly called Mexico's emigrants the unsung heroes of the republic (Durand 2004), only to be publicly countered by scholar Jorge Santibañez of Colegio de la Frontera Norte, who called them "actors in a national tragedy" (quoted in Thompson 2006). Immigrants undertake a perilous and risky journey, navigating unfamiliar and challenging job markets and social service landscapes. In spite of their resourcefulness, when migrants begin a family, they are sometimes accused of milking the system by the native-born. These conflicting interpretations of the efforts immigrants make to arrive in the United States and to work and live there affect them as they go about making decisions about whether to stay or go or when to start a family. The pregnancy stories of Mexican immigrant women cannot be separated from their immigration stories and their overall project, as immigrants, to improve their lot in life.

As such, the stories women tell about when, how, and why they started a family, the practices in which they engage during pregnancy, their birth experiences, and their reflections on all of these events never exist in a vacuum. On the contrary, they are embedded in and show discursive markings of broad societal trends, events, and pressures. Thus, the personal decision to try to become pregnant or to proceed with a pregnancy cannot be separated from a family's immigration stories, their background, their perception of the welcome their child is likely to receive by kin and the larger community, and more. In this book, I explore those interwoven stories, and although my focus is specifically on the experiences of Mexican immigrant women during pregnancy and childbirth, the relevance of these experiences to their lives in general is evident. Further, I contextualize their experiences within a larger economic and political context where powerful discourses circulate about these women and their families, discourses with which they must contend.

This study examines the irony that Mexican-born women are often eagerly complicit with models of care offered in public prenatal settings, even though such care may unravel the web of protective practices that promote healthy pregnancies. In prenatal clinics and social workers' offices, immigrant mothers are instructed in certain kinds of behaviors and postures based on their risk profile, socioeconomic status, and also prevailing attitudes about immigrants and their consumption of public resources. The intersection of medical care with immigration-specific ideas, attitudes, and experiences offers insight into the decline of the healthful, protective self-care practices that many Mexican immigrant women bring with them. Central to this project are both the enthusiasm many immigrant women have for what they perceive to be a technologically superior, modern health care system and the role accessing that system plays in their stories of immigration aspiration.

The findings of this study challenge some existing perceptions about the ways that immigrant families approach the idea of starting a family in the United States. In some of the negative discourses surrounding Mexican immigrants and immigration, immigrants are depicted as draining public resources and taking advantage of or gaming the system to gain free or reduced-cost health care, U.S. citizenship for their children, and welfare. Contrary to conservative pundits and other restrictionists' assumptions about families striving to have an "anchor baby" (Federation for American Immigration Reform 2009), who would establish an undocumented family's legitimacy and eventual eligibility for regularization of their status,[5] many families reported being deeply ambivalent about having children in the United States. When they decide to start a family, immigrants negotiate a complex terrain of services and manage conflicting advice from kin, friends, agencies, and health care providers about how to care for themselves and their babies.

Mexican immigrant women are perceived by many prenatal care providers to enter the public health care system well-equipped to have healthy babies. This positive characterization, which emerged in interviews with prenatal care providers in this study, contrasts with some of the characterizations of Mexican immigrants, and especially Mexican immigrant mothers, that circulate in the U.S. media and popular discourses. Although negative discourses surrounding immigrant women and their fertility infrequently enter directly into the prenatal care encounter, providers and patients are not immune to what anthropologist Leo Chavez calls the "biopolitics of immigration" (2008, 90). Assumptions they have about one another inevitably affect their interactions. Although condescending or inadequate care of immigrant women may often be simply a result of limited time and resources, it is a public health priority to disentangle the discourses surrounding immigrants from the treatment they receive (see also Wailoo, Livingston, and Guarnaccia 2006). When Mexican immigrant women access public prenatal care, they enter a system in which their prior knowledge about self-care in pregnancy and childbirth is often displaced, and they are instructed to behave as particular kinds of needy patients. These processes may ultimately undermine the protective and healthful habits and attitudes with which they entered the system. It is important to trace some of the ways this displacement occurs. It is my contention that these processes go a long way toward explaining the perinatal advantage of recent immigrant women and its decline with increased duration in the United States.

This book explores the ways that women reconcile these tumultuous currents, with an eye to determining how it is that many beneficial practices and knowledge are lost. In the process of being received and treated not as aspiring strivers but as high-risk, needy welfare recipients, Mexican immigrant women may leave behind modes of self-care in pregnancy; this process has a negative impact on their experiences of pregnancy and childbirth, on their own health and that of their children.

In this book, I identify some of the prime sites in which negotiations over care, knowledge, and attitudes take place, toward the goals of preserving the healthful practices with which many immigrant women enter the public health care system and of sharing that wealth with other recipients and providers of care.

Theoretical Framework

Anthropological attention to reproduction has generated a rich body of work on the production of biomedical hegemony in prenatal care settings. Authoritative knowledge, produced and monopolized by prenatal care providers in institutional contexts, has been argued to systematically "dislodge women's confidence in embodied knowledge" (Browner and Press 1996, 141). Brigitte Jordan has elaborated the concept of authoritative knowledge to trace the rise in biomedical approaches to childbirth (1993, 1997; see also Davis-Floyd and Sargent 1997; Hays 1996). She notes of authoritative knowledge that "it is important to realize that to identify a body of knowledge as authoritative speaks, for us as analysts, in no way to the correctness of that knowledge. Rather, the label 'authoritative' is intended to draw attention to its status within a particular social group and to the work it does in maintaining the group's definition of morality and rationality. The power of authoritative knowledge is not that it is correct, but that it counts" (Jordan 1997, 58).

This process occurs within the field referred to as the "technocratic model" (Davis-Floyd 1992) or "technomedicine": "a system of health care that objectifies the patient, mechanizes the body, and exalts practitioner over patient in a status hierarchy that attributes authoritative knowledge only to those who know how to manipulate the technology and decode the information it provides" (Davis-Floyd and Sargent 1997, 8). This book contributes to medical anthropology's understandings of authoritative knowledge and techno- or biomedicine, but it also can be read outside of that field within the study of racialization, immigrant assimilation, transnationalism, and public health research.

The ways that immigrant women receive messages about what they should do during pregnancy and childbirth and the response they have to those messages can be interpreted within critical analyses of reproduction. At the same time, these messages and immigrants' responses to them are part of their immigration stories. Although medical anthropologists have amply documented the ways that authoritative knowledge offers hard-to-refuse mandates about pregnancy care with which all expecting women contend, the reception of these mandates by immigrant women is arguably even more fraught. Not only does the knowledge of prenatal care providers come stamped with the trappings of credibility and authority, it is part of the very package of improved life circumstances that women hoped to access when they migrated in the first place. For many women, moving to New York City is viewed as an opportunity to better their lives and to access superior health care, resources, and opportunities for themselves and their children. Their initiation into what they often perceive as a superior system is slowly—if ever—perceived as a dehumanizing, humiliating, or damaging experience, even while women frequently report unsatisfying prenatal care, labor, and delivery experiences.

Drawing on Angela Valenzuela's work (1999) on subtractive schooling, I posit that ultimately what patients are offered is subtractive health care, a model for provisioning prenatal care that strips away and induces women themselves to shed the protective practices that have enabled them to have positive outcomes in the years immediately following their migration. The practices that epidemiologists and other scholars report as the "cultural advantage" of Mexican immigrant women during pregnancy and childbirth are inseparable from a legacy of poverty and what they view as "backward," home-based health care, which they enthusiastically discard within projects of self-improvement and aspirations to modernity. Here, we have a different kind of paradox, in which "health care" can lead to ill health, and healthful practices are willfully, even happily, left behind.

Research Methods

This is a multisited ethnographic research study that employs several qualitative methods.[6] The study employed ethnographic research methods, including participant observation, surveys, and life-history interviews, as well as quantitative analysis of individual medical records, public vital statistics, and census data. Research for this book was completed in various sites in New York City and, briefly, in Mexico. In New York City (n = 102), research was conducted at a major public hospital's prenatal clinic in Manhattan and at a community-service organization in Queens, New York; in addition the snowball method was used to contact participants. In Mexico (n = 6), research occurred in both rural and urban settings in Oaxaca and Puebla states. Research was conducted over two years, from 2006 to 2008, with one- to four-month-long intensive periods in each location; informal interviews occurred over a longer period.

In all, approximately one hundred Mexican immigrant women participated in New York City: sixty-three formal interviews, nineteen anonymous surveys in a hospital setting, and twenty women interviewed in a community organization and as a result of snowball referrals from other participants. All but one of the women were immigrants, born in Mexico. One woman, a nineteen-year-old interviewed during her second pregnancy, was born in New York to Mexican immigrant patients. On average, women in the study migrated 4.5 years prior to our first interview. They had lived in the United States from three months to twenty-one years. The average age upon arrival was 20.7 years. A small number of women migrated as children (also known as the 1.5 generation). Research among Mexicans in New York City offers a snapshot of a recent immigrant community in which the first generation still overwhelmingly outnumbers the 1.5 and succeeding generations.

I conducted all interviews myself, but I was assisted in surveys by a woman I call Señora Mercedes, a member of the Mexican diplomatic mission to New York City who generously assisted me on a voluntary basis. She expressed a deep interest in the project and concern for her countrywomen as they made their lives in New York City, although she also was known to interject her opinions and interpretations into informal conversations we had with patients. In addition, about a dozen prenatal care providers were interviewed.

When women's partners, friends, or family members accompanied them to the prenatal visits, they were sometimes included in conversations upon the request of the pregnant patient; each of these women was also interviewed on another occasion by herself. For the most part, however, this book does not include the perspectives of men on pregnancy and childbirth. Although their views would have greatly enriched the project, it was not feasible given the design and the location.[7] Further, while the interviews included open-ended life histories, this project was not intended to address or include all aspects of the lives of its participants.

The longer life-history interviews were typically conducted over one or more sessions lasting approximately thirty minutes to one hour each but, in a few cases, as long as three hours. Women in the public hospital who volunteered to participate were invited to talk to the researcher while awaiting their prenatal care appointments. The interviews were conducted in the language of the interviewee's choice (only one woman chose English over Spanish), in a private room, designated the "research room," within the prenatal clinic. These interviews were constrained by the unpredictability of the patients' wait time. The researcher assured participants that they would not be required to spend any additional time beyond the wait time for their appointments. Further, regular interview sessions were kept deliberately short out of consideration for the discomfort some women in late pregnancy feel when sitting for long periods. Many women engaged in multiple conversations with the researcher over subsequent clinic visits. More open-ended and longer conversations were also conducted in the labor and delivery ward, recovery rooms, and outside the hospital in a Queens community organization, as well as in women's homes. The open-ended interview schedule allowed participants to frame their life histories and to avoid any topics they felt uncomfortable discussing.

In addition to pregnant women and mothers, more than a dozen health care professionals were interviewed or accompanied in their clinical practice, including midwives, obstetricians, nutritionists, social workers, nurses, and physician's assistants in the public hospital in New York, as well as a general practitioner, two midwives, and a botanist in the Rio Blanco neighborhood of Oaxaca City; Ixtlán de Juárez, Oaxaca; and San Antonio Texcala and Zapotitlán Salinas, Puebla. All but one of the participating practitioners were women. These interviews and participant observation were aimed at identifying some of the opinions and perceptions of health care providers toward the patients in their care. Prenatal care providers in New York City revealed opinions and knowledge about Mexican patients that in some cases defied and in other cases confirmed the characterizations that are prominent in media and popular discourse. Further, providers' considered opinions, perceptions, and experiences with Mexican patients were often more accessible in interviews and extended conversations than they were in observations of clinical encounters where demands on providers' time often precluded reflection or explanation. Many of the providers in New York City were knowledgeable about research on the birth-weight paradox and eager to share with me their explanations for what is frequently described as an epidemiological mystery. Further, many of the immigrant mothers I interviewed described changing their practices or choosing not to reveal their behavior to their providers in responses to the anticipated opinions and preferences of providers. Although the emphasis in this study is on women's practices and experiences, I viewed it as important for the providers also to have an opportunity to share their views. In Mexico, practitioners were interviewed with the aim of learning about the political economy of prenatal care and childbirth in immigrant-sending communities. Further, they were asked to give their perspective on practices particular to the region that are associated with prenatal care and childbirth, including the use of herbs and thermal baths.

Ethnographic research allows the researcher to listen attentively, what João Biehl calls "disciplined listening" (2005:11), to the ways in which participants describe, narrate, and make sense of their lives. The very act of building a story requires elements of metanarrative: contextualization within the social, political, and economic events of the day; temporal and spatial perspectives; sequencing and logic. By listening to women's experiences with pregnancy and childbirth, I looked for clues to the protective practices in which recent immigrant women engage and the circumstances in which they decide to leave behind some of these practices.

Ethics

Current federal guidelines governing research with human subjects define pregnant women, but not undocumented immigrants, as a "vulnerable population." Nonetheless, in this and previous research projects with similar populations, I have been concerned that respondents were at greater risk because of the possible revelation of their potential undocumented immigrant status than because of any other factor in their participation. This study required approval by institutional review boards at the following places: the university that employed me over the first part of the research phase, the university that has employed me for the second part of the research phase to the present, the hospital, and the school of medicine affiliated with the hospital. I obtained a Certificate of Confidentiality from the National Institutes of Health that meant that I could not be compelled to reveal the identities or identifying characteristics of participants in any legal proceedings. Even so, I worried that my access to participants' personal data, including medical records, imposed a tremendous burden of responsibility. My research protocol followed very closely the norms guiding hospital-based research, and thus visits to the homes of participants recruited in the hospital were not a planned part of the study.[8] Accustomed to being barraged with consent forms and federal privacy-guideline brochures and forms in the hospital, patients rarely seemed discomfited by my formal consent procedure or inquisitiveness.[9] If I had then suggested that I might wish to accompany them on their daily rounds or to visit them at home, I would have posed a risk to their privacy as well as jeopardized their trust. Therefore, my research with prenatal care patients was rather more formal and constrained than my research with participants in other settings. Although this procedure limited the depth of my knowledge about their lives, it may have reassured them that their privacy would be protected.

When patients came to the hospital for a prenatal visit, they were given the opportunity to self-identify as Mexican and over the age of sixteen and were extended an invitation to participate in the study.[10] Those who chose to learn more visited me in the research office, located in the prenatal clinic, where I explained the study and offered them the opportunity to participate. Those who accepted were read a consent statement and asked to sign it if they agreed to participate. Those who did not have time or interest in participating in a life-history interview were offered the opportunity to complete an anonymous survey. Patients were given the option to deepen their participation by inviting me to the labor and delivery department when they came in to deliver their babies. A few patients chose to do this, even though my consent procedure and research protocol required that they contact me and prohibited me from following up with them over the phone. Conducting research directly in the prenatal care setting, then, gave me an only limited view of some participants' lives, but this drawback was compensated for by the incredible richness of material gained through observing firsthand the prenatal care encounter.

In this book, all research participants are identified by pseudonyms. All the pseudonyms were randomly selected from a database, including the names of participants in the study and some of those of their relatives, friends, and children, for greater fidelity to patterns of naming than if the pseudonyms were entirely researcher-selected.

I have chosen to use a pseudonym for the hospital in which I conducted research, Manhattan Hospital Center. Although my research began and ended there with respect and admiration for the efforts of Manhattan Hospital to offer midwifery and birthing-center options to uninsured and Medicaid-insured patients, I felt the privacy of the participants in the study would be better protected by not revealing the name of the hospital. I came away from my research convinced that Manhattan is a public institution comprising individuals who work tirelessly to offer the most innovative, comprehensive, and humane care they can in a context of oversubscription and continual underfunding that has become increasingly acute (especially since the privatization of Medicaid by New York State Governor George Pataki in 2000). For that reason, although I recount in the text many moments when the hospital failed to live up to its ideals, I concur with many of the patients I interviewed there that it is the best the city has to offer.

New York City's Mexican Population

Scholars call the growth since 1990 of the Mexican population in New York City "accelerated," meaning that it has taken less than a generation for the community to grow from the original "pioneer" migrants to comprising so many people that nearly every family in some rural Mexican towns can name a member living in New York City (Cortes 2003). Although in 1990 as few as 53,000 Mexicans had migrated to New York City, in 2010 that number was at least 319,263, a nearly sixfold growth (U.S. Census 2010), which was only showing signs of slowing with the financial crisis of 2008–2010. The Mexican Consulate estimates that 50 percent of the Mexican-origin population in New York City may be undocumented. Of all Latino groups in New York City, Mexicans have the highest percentage of immigrants, 63–70 percent (Rivera Batiz 2002, 5; U.S. Census Bureau 2005), an indication of the recentness of migration and the still nascent second generation. Of Mexican women who gave birth in New York City, 96.8 percent were foreign-born in 2000. That number fell significantly by 2008 but remained very high at 91.2 percent (Begier et al. 2010; New York City Department of Health and Mental Hygiene 2008).

Although the Mexican population in New York City includes highly educated professionals, business people, and students who originate from all states in Mexico, this study is focused on consumers of public prenatal care, a subset of the larger Mexican population. Consumers of public prenatal care are less likely than others to have private medical insurance or the resources to pay for private medical care and are more likely to receive publicly subsidized prenatal care. The sample here thus includes a greater than representative number of low-income migrants from poor, rural areas of Mexico, many of whom entered the United States without authorization. This population is not representative of the broader Mexican immigrant population.

Although migratory status was not an object of inquiry, it became apparent in interviews that most of the women included in this study were living in the United States without authorization. The more recent a person's migration, the greater the likelihood that he or she entered without authorization. Further, undocumented status was indicated by the respondents' descriptions of their arrival in the United States and their use of public prenatal care, for which undocumented immigrants are eligible, but not of food stamps, for which they are not. Further, given the demographic characteristics of the Mexican and the undocumented immigrant populations in New York City and my location in immigrant-serving institutions, it is likely that the population included in the study included a greater proportion of Mexican immigrants who were undocumented than did the city as a whole. Thus, although the study revealed much about immigrant women's experiences in public prenatal care, it revealed even more about the specific experiences of undocumented Mexican women. This fact is of both sociological and theoretical importance. The particular political, social, and discursive space occupied by women who are undocumented immigrants in the national polity is an inseparable component of their experiences as mothers. Further, William McCarthy and his colleagues (2005), among others, have emphasized the importance of taking into consideration immigration status when examining ethnic differences in health status (also Harley 2004).

The flow of new migrants from Mexico to New York City is coupled with a steep birth rate. In 2005, the number of births to Mexican mothers was 2.5 times the average among Latino groups, and more than nine times the birth rate for the city as a whole (138 per 1000, versus 15.3 for the city, Bergad 2008, 4; Ruíz-Navarro 2009 asserts that the rate for New York is actually the highest of all states at 165.9 per 1000).[11] Mexican mothers had more babies (8,474) than all but three other groups: African Americans (17,292), Puerto Ricans (10,229), and Dominicans (9,855) (New York City Department of Health and Mental Hygiene 2008), even while Mexicans constitute only 10 percent of the Latino population and 3 percent of the total population of the city (U.S. Census 2005). More women who gave birth in New York City in 2007 were born in Mexico, 6.3 percent, than in any other country after the United States, an indicator of the large percentage of Mexican mothers who are immigrants (97 percent) and the high birth rates of this immigrant group (New York City Department of Health and Mental Hygiene 2008).

Outline of Book

The remaining chapters of this book examine the experiences of Mexican immigrant women with pregnancy and childbirth in New York City. In Chapter 2, I begin with a look at the "immigrant experience": the ways that being an immigrant implies, for many women, an aspirational stance and an eagerness to better one's lot in life, a process initiated when they leave their hometowns. This enthusiasm to ensure that their own and their children's life chances are superior to those in their hometowns often implies a willingness to adopt the features of what they perceive to be the fast-paced, modern lifestyle associated with New York. Although they do not wish to leave behind what they call their "culture," they usually came to the United States with a project, abstractly defined as a project to "improve" or "overcome" themselves and their life chances, or *superarse*. The attitudes and expectations associated with this kind of project are characteristic of the actual journey of migrating to the United States and beginning a life there and also have an impact on women's work-force participation, decisions about when and where to start a family, and the family size they consider ideal. They also shape the ways women engage the agencies of the state, social service agencies, community organizations, and the individuals and groups with whom they share their lives. These aspects of their immigrant narratives are inseparable not only temporally but also discur-sively from their approach to pregnancy care and child-rearing. In this chapter, I also discuss the growth of anti-immigrant discourses in the United States, especially immigrant women's fertility and their babies as targets for special ire. These discourses, which are prevalent in mass media as well as in local interactions, color the decisions that families make and their perception of the social context in which they plan to raise their children.

In Chapter 3, I look at what women describe as typical pregnancy care and childbirth experiences in their hometowns, as well as at the changing social, medical, and economic landscape of prenatal care and birth in Mexico. In this chapter, I listen attentively to what women say about their own and their female kin's experiences with pregnancy and childbirth "allá en el pueblo," back home. I describe the vast repertoire of care practices for pregnant and post-partum mothers by midwives and female kin that many women describe as customary in their communities of origin. And, by enriching interviews with pregnant women and mothers in New York City with data gained through research in the regions of Mexico from which some of them migrated, I am able to trace the ways birth practices have changed in Mexico at the same time that the lives of these immigrants have changed. Their descriptions of "typical" childbirth experiences in many cases date to 2000 or before, the period preced-ing their migration. In the intervening years, the federal government has pene-trated much of the countryside with publicly funded clinics and a regime of certification that have virtually eliminated traditional midwifery in many rural communities. Thus, although many women describe spatial contrast, contrast-ing "here" and "there," talking to some of their sisters, mothers, and birth atten-dants in their hometowns reveals also some temporal dissonance, in which the norms women remember surrounding pregnancy and childbirth simply are no longer dominant. Pregnancy and birth practices are in a period of transformation and contention as immigrants come to the United States but also as their hometowns are subject to an enormous public health campaign by the Mexican federal government amid narratives of progress and modernity.

In Chapter 4, I look at the birth experiences of Mexican immigrant women in public care settings in New York City. I follow the ways that women describe their experiences, and listen to their joys and frustrations. I trace the predominant path by which women access public prenatal care, through Medicaid eligibility, and follow the ways that establishing and maintaining access requires women to submit to an intrusive and often coercive regime established by social workers, nutritionists, nurses, doctors, and sometimes midwives.

In Chapter 5, I identify the protective and beneficial practices engaged in by Mexican immigrant women during pregnancy and discuss when, how, and why these practices begin to fall away. In spite of a reputation for being stoic and docile, Mexican immigrant women frequently hold contrarian views toward routine interventions and protocols in prenatal care and labor and delivery. I examine how they reconcile their openness and enthusiasm about some aspects of public prenatal care with their own embodied experiences of being able, without a great deal of supervision and intervention, to give birth to healthy babies.

In Chapter 6, I conclude by analyzing the story about pregnancy and childbirth told in these pages as an immigration story. Using citizenship theory and theories about social reproduction and race, I look at the ways that current immigration law, processes of racialization, and conflicting notions about the eligibility of immigrants for citizenship affect the birth experiences of immigrant women. I identify the life-cycle events of pregnancy and childbirth generally, and the prenatal care encounter specifically, as key sites for the clash and negotiation of ideas about rights, entitlements, human worth, and the public good; and I give prescriptions for improving the encounter between immigrant women and health care institutions in the United States.

Chapter 2

Immigrant Aspirations and the Decisions Families Make

Claudia did not wish to migrate from her home in Castillotla, Puebla. Nevertheless, her partner, who had been in the United States before, thought they should, and, with a baby on the way, she said, "Uno piensa en los dos, no sólo en uno" [You think about the two of you, not just yourself]. She had a terrible time crossing the border in Arizona. She was returned to Mexico seven times by the border patrol. She worried about the immediate risks posed by her crossing, and she also worried about going through the remainder of her pregnancy far from her mother and mother-in-law. Over the phone, they attempted to care for Claudia the way they would if she were still in Castillotla. But, in New York City, Claudia said she and her partner were together and they could "sacar a la familia adelante" [pull the family ahead].[1] Even though Claudia did not come to the United States because of personal ambition, her migration was part of a larger project, calculated to enable her and her partner to improve their lives and that of the child who was on the way. Separation from her family, the rupture of the networks of women who would have cared for her and the baby during pregnancy and after birth, even the economic expense of crossing and then settling as a couple in a costly city were secondary to the overall project of unity as a family and a project to better their circumstances.

Rosario had her first child in San Pablo, outside of Apizaco, Tlaxcala, Mexico. Left by her husband, she lived with her father, who helped maintain her. When a sister died of cancer, still grieving, she decided to leave everything behind and migrate to New York: "Decidí quedarme un tiempo aquí para realizarme" [I decided to stay for a while to fulfill myself]. Now, five years later, she is expecting her second child and is happy. Her partner, she says, supports her, and, she explains, "Me siento capaz" [I feel capable].

Columba came because of economic need: "No había que comer" [There was nothing to eat]. She left her four children with her mother in Ocuapa, near Chilpancingo de Bravo, Puebla, and crossed the border with a coyote her partner hired.[2] She works in a factory, sewing. Nayeli came from Acatlán de Osorio, Puebla, explaining, "Bueno, como siempre, este . . . querer trabajar, salir adelante y tener un porvenir" [Well, like always . . . wanting to work, to get ahead and have a future].

Although each of these women came because of individual, sometimes tragic, circumstances, their stories share a common thread. Each had the desire to better her life circumstances, a process often referred to in Spanish by those in this study with the noun *superación* or with the verb *superarse*. To migrate is a dramatic rupture that is also often seen as a means to proactively alter one's path. *Superarse*—literally, to surpass oneself, or better oneself—is the answer frequently given to the question "¿Por qué te viniste?" [Why did you come?]: "Para superarme."

Douglas Massey and Magaly Sánchez identify five main categories of motivation for international migration, each of which was well represented in this study's sample: economic conditions at origin, economic conditions at destination, network connections, violence at origin, and family reunification (2010, 39). Although their projects are not always successful and some come to view their migration as a "bad investment," as one interviewee put it, the locating of their migration within a larger aspirational frame influences immigrants' approach to life in the United States.

Although some migrate as a youthful rite of passage, for others migration is a last resort, a costly, risky venture in which the stakes are extremely high. In turn, typically not only the migrant herself has high hopes for her sojourn in New York; migrants have an average of four people they have left behind who will depend on their remittances (Suárez Orozco 2009). María Islas (2010) writes about the "transnational dreams" of migrants and the families that stay behind, asserting that family members who never migrate increasingly stake their aspirations on the fortunes of those who leave for the United States. As a result, as trying and dangerous as their crossing may be and despite the difficulties they often face in establishing themselves in the United States, migrants frequently adopt a posture of openness and enthusiasm toward life in a new country. Islas argues that through practices of transnational dreaming, people think about the future in ways that produce subjectivity in the present. In this way, for those who migrate, the future in some important sense is now.

In the small and large acts of migrating to and making a life in New York City migrants perform their imagined future selves even as they contend with various practical limitations on the realization of these versions of themselves. Arjun Appadurai takes as central the "everyday cultural practice through which the work of the imagination is transformed" (1996, 9). I do the same. How does an imaginative stance, a posture inclined toward future, modern versions of themselves shape immigrants' responses to the difficulties they face?

In this chapter, I trace the production of discourses of superación and analyze the ways that these discourses enable particular postures toward life in the United States. I situate these discourses within the larger context in which immigrants migrate, which includes their reasons for leaving their hometowns and their reasons for choosing New York as a destination. I also examine the emergent nativist and restrictionist discourses in the United States that scapegoat immigrants, and in particular Mexican immigrant women, as profligate breeders whose out-of-control fertility threatens U.S. prosperity, security, and national identity. To what degree are the interactions of Mexican immigrant families with their neighbors, educators, medical personnel, and others affected by these discourses? How do families contend with these attitudes as they go about making their lives and trying to offer their children the best possible futures?

Superación

This section focuses on the production of narratives of aspiration among would-be migrants in Mexico and immigrants already living in New York City. The impulse of parents to provide a better childhood for their children than what they experienced is a widespread motivation for migration (Hellman 2008; Lee 2008) regardless of whether migrants leave their children behind with relatives, take them along to their destination, or have not yet had children. Migration is at the same time the result of and the perceived solution to a truncated opportunity structure in many rural communities as well as in urban peripheries in Mexico.

Within narratives of superación, we can trace certain postures and attitudes that are activated in certain locations and interactions surrounding pregnancy and childbirth. Joan Scott writes that "it is not individuals who have experiences, but subjects who are constituted through experience" (Scott 1992, 26; also Wailoo, Livingston, and Guarnaccia 2006, 2). Valentina Napolitano traces the ways middle-class residents of Guadalajara appropriate modernity, seeing urban landscapes as an "important terrain for understanding how modernity and its failure are reinscribed, reimagined, and reproduced" in the "local cultural practices of modernity" (2002, 14). In similar fashion, Jennifer Hirsch writes that people use intimate relationships to act out modern gendered identities (2003, 12). Drawing on Judith Butler's work on gender as performance and on other feminist theory, these scholars examine ways that structure and agency intersect in the realm of the imagination, the performed articulation of possible selves that occurs within cross-cutting processes of subjectification. Crossing the border and taking up new lives in the United States, immigrant women, and especially undocumented immigrant women, are engaged in dynamic and at times brutal processes of "self making and being made," as described by Aihwa Ong (1996, 737). They work to articulate imagined selves by seeking to make strategic improvements over their lives in Mexico and over the lives to which they compare their own: those of their mothers and sisters. Although even the most idealistic immigrants are rarely under any illusions that they will quickly or easily strike it rich in *el norte*, they measure the worthiness of their investment in a migration project in incremental and metonymic alterations in their quality of life and security. In this fashion, consumption of health care becomes a measure of social capital that marks the distance traveled from hometowns in which most migrants describe not having access to affordable, modern biomedical care (see Viladrich 2003).[3] Keith Wailoo, Julie Livingston, and Peter Guarnaccia refer to the importance of health care in some narratives of migration as "the magnetic appeal of America's high-technology medicine" (2006, 4).

Further, immigrant women in this study described their efforts to cultivate relationships with their children and partners based on mutual appreciation, respect, and love. Instead of viewing family size as an aspect of life outside their control, many immigrant women describe elaborate negotiations, calculations, and considerations invested in building the right-sized and right-timed family in which everyone's needs can be well met. Their agency in this respect is consistent with Hirsch's findings regarding companionate marriage, family size, and contraception use among Mexican immigrants in Atlanta, Georgia (2003). In contrast to some of the common assumptions about Mexican immigrants' approach to starting a family, this study revealed the reluctance that many families have toward bearing and raising children in the United States, the efforts they make to limit and delay pregnancy, and the ways they manage their fertility.

Characterization and Reception of Migrants in New York City

Choosing to migrate to the United States is a weighty decision. Since the early 1990s, an increasing number of immigrants from Mexico have chosen the

New York area as their destination. Migrants come for many reasons: economic need, to study, to follow a romantic partner, family reunification, and on a whim. Striking out for a new country is, by definition, an aspirational act. Except in rare instances of coerced migration, virtually all immigrants have a faint or pronounced hope that migration will improve their life chances by enabling them to achieve something back home or to start a new chapter in their destination. This aspirational stance colors all encounters and interactions. Talk of this drive of new immigrants is one of the dominant narratives of New York City: "greenhorns" and starry-eyed dreamers who arrive on the city's hardened streets to make new lives; even Frank Sinatra sang about it. Impressions of Mexican immigrants as hard-working, driven, humble, family-oriented, and more can be heard around the city. Understanding the interactions of this recent group of immigrants with people and agencies in the city requires not only comprehension of the context from which they are migrating but also of the ways that their desire for superación imbues their posture toward the events and opportunities of life in New York City.

As the Mexican population has grown, struggles over migrants' representation, reception, and assimilation have become increasingly acute. Discourses about New York's character as an immigrant city where anyone has a chance and everyone is welcome clash with emergent strands of xenophobia, which became pronounced with the economic downturn in 2008 and heated national debates about immigration reform and undocumented immigration. Although Mexicans in the city were perceived in the 1980s and 1990s largely as "model" immigrants in many employment sectors as well as by some public service providers (Hellman 2008; Smith 2005), their growing numbers and anxiety about their supposed impact on wages and their consumption of public benefits have caused some decidedly anti-Mexican sentiments and violence to bubble to the surface in New York neighborhoods.[4] Processes of racialization, amply documented by social scientists, bombard this new population, determining where its members "belong" and should end up: positively viewed as model immigrants or disparaged as invaders and a drain on resources.[5] Of course, model-immigrant status implies its own violence and exclusion, even while it affords some privileges to those so designated. Model-immigrant status leads to implicit—and sometimes explicit—denigration of others and is also often premised on stereotypes about behavior, culture, and practices, stereotypes that may be limited, biased, and stifling. For Mexicans in New York, the moniker "hardworking," often accompanied by such adjectives as "docile" and "stoic," can lead to labor exploitation of those who struggle to meet employer expectations and reprobation of those who defy it by, say, asking for a fair wage or safety gear (see De Genova and Ramos-Zayas 2003). Nonetheless, Mexican immigrants frequently remarked in interviews during this and previous studies that their nationality was favorably viewed by employers—a status that surely causes no small amount of ire on the part of other immigrants who may be negatively compared with them.

Negative characterizations of Mexicans have been more prevalent in historical receiving communities in the southwestern United States than in New York City, with immigrants viewed as repositories for anxieties about a whole range of issues from the globalization of the economy to the increasing relevance of the Spanish language, but these characterizations are on the rise in New York. Even in supposedly sanitized and ideologically neutral environments like public hospitals and schools, Mexican immigrants receive mixed messages about their roles as parents, their culture, their children, and their eligibility for both the material and the intangible benefits of belonging.

Public prenatal clinics and hospitals are locations for some of the most exciting and emotional interactions and events in immigrant families' lives but are also a prime site for socialization and racialization. Even though health care providers frequently hold progressive political and social views and express outwardly pro-immigrant sentiments, they serve as gatekeepers, administering access to public benefits and schooling patients in acceptable and appropriate behaviors. Further, in the absence of a care protocol that allows time to hear immigrant patients speak about their hopes, dreams, experiences, and wisdom, public hospitals can fall into patterns of racialization even as professionals within them often harbor progressive values and deep respect for their patients.

In the waiting areas, exam rooms, and labor and delivery wards of public hospitals a great deal of work is done—not only the work of caring for pregnant women and delivering their babies but also the work of social reproduction: the formation of certain kinds of subjects. Although each individual patient and provider has distinct perspectives and experiences, trends can be discerned in which immigrant patients reconcile their aspirations to a constrained arena of possible identities. The organization of space, time, and resources in these environments does not permit a limitless range of individual expressions of knowledge, experience, and desire, but requires patients to present themselves as self-sufficient or needy, compliant or not, educated or ignorant. The repercussions of these processes of categorization are immeasurable. The quality and type of care they receive may be based on these characterizations. It is one of the contentions of this book that the initial taxonomy shapes a lifetime of interactions with the state and its agencies. The posture and positioning available to immigrant women in prenatal care interactions have not only a formative role in shaping the content and form of the benefits and treatment they receive but clear health consequences as well. In short, turning Mexican immigrant women from strivers into needy welfare recipients is bad medicine.

Mirna migrated to New York from Cholula, Puebla, ten years before I interviewed her at Manhattan Hospital. She told me that over the course of three pregnancies, for all of which she received care at Manhattan Hospital, she radically changed her eating habits and also acquired information that she used to adjust her approach to parenting in ways she perceived to be beneficial. In Mexico, she told me, people eat fried, fatty foods, including tamales and tacos. She said these are not healthy foods and that in the hospital she was advised by a nutritionist to cut tortillas out of her diet. She also learned to eat roasted meats and chicken and to increase her consumption of vegetables. She said she began to eat almost entirely low-fat foods, drank a lot of milk, and stopped using sugar. She proudly reported to me that she did not gain any extra weight during her pregnancies. She went on to describe an overall approach to life that involved setting herself apart from the way she used to be, the manner of life she associated with her hometown and with her compatriots. She proudly told me that she did not receive any public benefits, noting that this was the only way that undocumented immigrants might hope to demonstrate worthiness for future immigration reform. She said she and her family share an apartment with Ecuadorans because "they treat you better; one cannot rely on one's own countrymen." She described the ways she and her husband raised their children in what she called a more wholesome environment than that of other families she knew, including spending free time together as a family. She also said she tried to read a lot while pregnant so that her children would be intelligent.

Mirna's approach to parenting was a reflection of a confluence of influences and contextual factors, shaped by her acceptance of what she viewed as the superior approaches to diet, child-rearing, family life, and pregnancy available to her in the United States. Especially in her many critiques of other parents whom she knew, she characterized her role as a mother as proactively carving the best path she could for her children based on knowledge, practices, and attitudes garnered from the nutritionist's office, the materials she read, her exposure to people from other ethnic groups, and more. Mirna seemed to seek to actively demonstrate her own "evolution" as a mother, proud of her ability to flexibly adapt to new information and reject practices that she felt were given undue respect by others simply because they were specific to their country or culture: "tradition." In this way, Mirna's approach to migration was not simply about improving her family's economic or educational future but about becoming a better person. Grace Chang found in her research that negative societal attitudes about immigrants' putative consumption of public resources are so prevalent that they are sometimes internalized and reproduced by immigrants themselves (2000, 37; also Gutiérrez 2008, 121; Pease Chock 1996). Mirna here reproduces dominant and pejorative links between consumption of welfare and moral failure.

Although many would dispute her characterization of Mexican food as invariably fatty and unhealthy, there is nothing inherently wrong, according to most medical recommendations, with the adaptations and adjustments Mirna made. Mirna and many other women I interviewed construct something of a binary in which the advice they obtain in the United States is viewed as superior and the practices they bring from home as inferior. This binary, although seldom so Manichean, can accelerate the widening of the gap between practices associated with "home" and "host" locales.

Anti-Immigrant Trends

The aspirational stance of immigrants is familiar to nonimmigrants in the United States. However, it has now been taken up by anti-immigrant activists and cast as a plot on the part of immigrants to take advantage—illegitimately, they say—of the benefits associated with membership in the nation. This attitude is evidenced by a rise in hate crimes against immigrants as well as by the increasing visibility of anti-immigrant organizations like the Minuteman Project.[6]

As public demonstrations in favor of immigration reform and legislative movement toward such reform have increased, so too has anti-immigrant sentiment, expressed in various ways through restrictionist, nativist, demographic, and other discourses. In some regions, tension over immigrants, especially undocumented Latino immigrants, is so high that it pervades virtually all discussions of politics and the public sphere. In 2010, public discussion of the issue of immigration reform reached a fervor with the passage of Arizona law SB 1070, requiring anyone suspected of being an undocumented resident to produce identity papers on request and also criminalizing unlawful presence in the state. This law prompted fears of racial profiling and other harassment of immigrants and of anyone who purportedly resembled an immigrant.[7]

Mexican Women's Fertility: Trojan Horse
of Conquest or Economic Salvation?

Anthropologist Leo Chavez describes the "Latino threat narrative" as the "dark matter surrounding public discourse. It's everywhere." He notes that it is manifest in its most extreme variety as paranoia about a "secret Mexican plan to take over the United States" (2008, 3; 2009). Chavez argues that within these narratives "the head of the invading army is the Trojan horse of reproduction: Mexican women's fertile bodies" (2009). Pregnant Mexican immigrants are perhaps the repository of more anxiety and tension than any other figures in the contemporary United States polity. Anti-immigrant sentiment seems to simmer around the issue of reproduction. Chavez traces how "new" nativist sentiments center on "reproduction—women and children—and [do] little to stop the production work of immigrant labor" (1997, 69). Chang, building on June Nash, similarly writes, "Global capital prefers to exploit women as producers, rather than reproducers. . . . Increasing immigrant women's production while limiting their reproduction facilitates utilizing immigrant women as expendable workers by ensuring that they will not bear more unwanted consumers or expand a population that has needs" (2000, 101; also Newton 2008, 26; Pease Chock 1996; Yuval-Davis and Werbner 1999, 23).

This use of women is nothing new. In fact, it is a typical consequence of colonial and postcolonial relations. As Laura Briggs writes, in reference to the United States's neocolonialist relationship to Puerto Rico in the early twentieth century, "Gender and women's bodies became a significant idiom in which colonial relations were negotiated" (2002, 70). This view is equally applicable to the contemporary neocolonial relationship between the United States as an economic center in the hemisphere and its neighbors to the south, which provide an increasing number of workers in low-wage sectors through both migration to the United States and reproduction by Latino immigrants within it. The industrialized North's demand for new workers, which until the economic recession that began in 2008 seemed insatiable, runs contrary to the anxieties among some residents of receiving nations about overpopulation and environmental degradation. Far from accidental or circumstantial, Chang calls the relationship between the North's demand for labor and the supply of undocumented workers from developing nations a product of social "engineering" designed to match low-wage workers with the employers that demand them (2000, 13). Briggs maps the production of social difference and racialization on women's bodies and the public health policies designed to regulate them. Much of Social Darwinian and Malthusian theories about poverty, overpopulation, environmental degradation, migration, and even geopolitical instability have been centered on the bodies and fertility of "third-world" women. These politicoscientific fields have provided an ostensibly "neutral" and science-based platform from which to critique poor women's fertility. As Briggs writes, "Over the course of four decades, the trope of the dangerous mother as the cause of poverty made its way, in both overseas development projects and domestic welfare policy, from liberal to neoconservative to neoliberal projects. . . . The status of the 'welfare queen' has sometimes differed from that of the mother of third world overpopulation but they continue to be in conversation with each other. What remains constant is the centrality of ideologies about women—victimized or dangerous—to provide the cause for policy intervention, and reproduction and sexuality to provide the core of a discourse of racial/national/class difference" (2002, 191).

Mexican women's fertility has been the subject of tremendous scrutiny in the United States, and that scrutiny only grows as immigration debates become increasingly heated. Elena Gutiérrez chronicles the process beginning a century ago by which "the hyper-fertile Mexican immigrant woman once again gained infamy as a social problem necessitating public action and governmental intervention" (Gutiérrez 2008, 110; also Milanich 2009, 24; Newton 2008).

Negative discourses about Mexican women's fertility produce powerful and pervasive ideas that receive their most elaborate development among nativists and restrictionists but that spill over into mainstream media and popular discourse, in part because of the efforts of a network of organizations sharing the same founders, boards of directors, funders, and objectives but different tactics and constituencies (Federation for American Immigration Reform, Numbers USA, and Center for Immigration Studies) (Sterling 2010). The anti-immigrant sentiments underlying these messages, often cloaked as concerns about population growth, the environment, and even Latin American poverty, make their way into the spaces of immigrant-serving institutions in places as ostensibly pro-immigrant as New York City and its public institutions. In this way, immigrants are constructed as a "social problem" (Gutiérrez 2008; Newton 2008, 34). In these constructions, Mexico, an underdeveloped "third-world" country, has rampant fertility and patriarchal social relations that ensure that women's only purpose is to serve as baby-making machines; as a result, they produce an excessively numerous population and an emigration problem. Thus, culturally and economically irresponsible and backward attitudes are seen to have produced the overpopulation, poverty, and economic degradation that drive migrants to the North, where they seek work. Once in the United States, still hyperfertile Mexican women are thought to drain the comparatively wealthy and benevolent state coffers of public resources without contributing their share through labor. Were they here only to work, they might be acceptable, but it is feared that the flow of people migrating to have babies will bankrupt the United States and turn it into the "third world." In these sorts of narratives, nativists and restrictionists try to argue that they are not racist, that they wish, rather, that Mexico—which is described as being run by elite oligarchs of European stock—would educate and create jobs for its people instead of keeping them down, exploited and backward, mired in a traditional, patriarchal, racist, and repressive society.[8]

The attitudes toward immigrant women who do a great deal of the caring work in the United States and yet are demonized as hyperfertile and ignorant baby machines are contradictory but make sense within the economic and political relationships between the United States and its neighbors, as well as between middle- and upper-class employers and immigrant women workers. This attitude is related to the notion of "stratified reproduction," developed by Shellee Cohen. Faye Ginsburg and Rayna Rapp sum up this idea as follows: "Stratified reproduction . . . describe[s] the power relations by which some categories of people are empowered to nurture and reproduce, while others are disempowered. . . . More broadly, who defines the body of the nation into which the next generation is recruited? Who is considered to be in that body, who is out of it? . . . Thus, put starkly, the concept of stratified reproduction helps us to see the arrangements by which some reproductive futures are valued while others are despised" (1995, 3). Nira Yuval-Davis and Pnina Werbner similarly write, "Women as mothers and citizens . . . are constructed as bearers of either negative or positive futures" (1999, 16).

Analyses like these assert that stratified reproduction and undocumented migration are features of a larger globalized economic system in which poor women of color are recruited to perform caring labor in the global North. In this way, declining birth rates are viewed as a sign of progress and civilization, enabling the fetishization of the child in elite sectors and the marginalization of or even the attribution of abject status to the children of the poor. No matter how few children immigrant mothers have, their children are always excessive, hindering their mothers' labor capacity, draining resources, and reasserting the humanity of their parents (an inconvenient reminder that serves to mitigate their exploitability). Chavez, further, writes, "The fertility of white women is not only normative, but they also possess 'subject status' which Jurgen Link defines as 'an autonomous, responsible, *quasi* juridical person of sound mind as in a legal subject.' In contrast, Latinas do not possess subject status as their behavior is viewed as irrational, illogical, chaotic, subject to tradition and superstition and therefore threatening" (2008, 74; also Pease Chock 1996).

We can invert these interpretations of Mexican and other Latina immigrant women's fertility: Latinas are having the babies that other women no longer have and are thus ensuring stability in the labor market and economic prosperity for future generations. Chavez explains this phenomenon as follows: "Would it be possible to make the following observation: the abnormally *low* fertility rates of white women are leading to demographic changes and increased pressure for immigration?" (2008, 110). The birth rate in the United States in fact steadily dropped over the previous century. Some interpret this drop as an inevitable feature of modernization. Simon Szreter, a critic of demographic-transition theory, describes this assumption as follows: "Although there was nothing historically inevitable in the process, in order to industrialize and modernize, a country must pass through the stages of demographic transition, with the appearance of fertility-controlling behavior marking the advent of a final stage, and the general spread of such behavior confirming successful sociocultural adjustment to the conditions of a modernized, economically developed nation" (1993, 662). But, as Szreter makes clear, fertility decline is attributable to multiple factors and is not at all inevitable. Nonetheless, the decline in fertility among the native-born population in the United States is often viewed as a sign of progress and modernity.[9] Fertility-decline measures are thus worn on women's backs, read as measures of their country's progress on a single teleological path toward development and modernity.

The labor market has continued to demand more workers than are being produced within the United States. Acquisition of a college degree has become more common and accessible than ever before, making the U.S. labor force, on average, better educated and more equipped for jobs in the so-called FIRE (finance, investment, real estate) industries, which drive the U.S. postmanufacturing economy (Wallace and Wallace 1998). Still, there are gaps at the top of the labor market (highly specialized technical fields, typically requiring a Ph.D.) as well as at the bottom (construction, service, agriculture) that are filled in increasing numbers by immigrants. Work visas are largely available only for the higher-end, specialized jobs, and thus it is likely that workers who fill lower-wage positions have entered the country without authorization. As journalist and conservative pundit Tamar Jacoby writes, an average of a million and a half new immigrants each year are absorbed into the U.S. economy, but only two-thirds of them are able to get visas; this situation generates an annual spillover of about a half-million illegal workers (2007).[10] To an ever-growing degree, the economic viability of the United States depends on the labor of immigrants and their children. Nevertheless, even though "immigration-reform" proposals typically allow some to regularize their status, they increase restrictions on nonworking adults and children, or, in other words, they "target reproduction of the immigrant labor force" (Chavez 1997, 66).

Some scholars hold that, in fact, unauthorized immigrant laborers and their children have enabled the United States to continue to grow economically since the early 1990s (Chang 2000; De Genova 2005, 2009; Dreby 2010; Holmes 2009; Sider 2003). This growth is subsidized in two ways. First, the nations that send migrants to the United States as workers are to a significant degree subsidizing U.S. economic growth. When a worker migrates as a young adult, his family, community, and nation have already invested in his health, education, and training.[11] Thus, poor communities in Mexico and elsewhere are subsidizing the growth of the U.S. labor force by producing strong, capable workers who lend the most productive years of their lives to the United States, perhaps returning to their home communities only to retire. The starkest expression of this model was seen prior to the militarization of the border (beginning in the mid-1990s). Typically a male head of household migrated alone and sent remittances back to provide for a spouse, children, and extended family in his home community. In this way, rural Mexican communities turned into "retirement homes and nurseries," as many analysts in Mexico describe it; they assumed all the expense of producing new generations of workers and of caring for them when they could no longer work. Sociologists Pierette Hondagneu-Sotelo and Ernestine Avila call this the "externalization of the cost of labor reproduction to Mexico and Central America" and "a dream come true" for restrictionists (1997, 568; also Pease Chock 1996). Over the course of a generation, many towns in Mexico became "dollarized," with family income measured only in remittances received from abroad (Alvarado 2010). These communities do not benefit from the productiveness of their most capable members, except in the form of their remittances, which are a smaller portion of the workers' productive capacity than what stays in the United States in the form of living expenses; sales, payroll, and property taxes; profits generated for their employers; and more. Chang argues that this arrangement is not coincidental and not a product of decontextualized "push" and "pull" factors but rather is "aimed at [a single] objective: to capture the labor of immigrant men and women separate from their human needs or those of their dependents" (2000, 11).

Second, since the increase in border militarization in the mid-1990s, increasing numbers of families of undocumented workers have decided to immigrate together or to have children in the United States, but they do so as part of a strategy of maximizing the labor-force participation of their working members. These families assume a greater responsibility than the average U.S. family for the expenses of child-rearing and raising a new generation of workers because of their presumed or actual exclusion from many of the benefits of citizenship (Chang 2000, 13; Passel 2005). They are ineligible for many forms of public assistance and financial aid, less likely to hold health insurance, less likely to receive prenatal care and wellness care, less likely to attend well-performing schools, less likely to graduate (Passel 2005). It is also arguable that this situation is not accidental; processes of racialization and discrimination produce an undereducated and underskilled generation of new workers who are more likely to take jobs at lower wage rates.

If "deportability" enables undocumented workers to fill the most exploited niches in the U.S. economy to the advantage of their employers and the economy in general (De Genova 2005; also Newton 2008), racialization and the perpetuation of inequality for their U.S.-born children—who are not deportable—are the only ways to ensure the continuation of an exploitable class if border securitization succeeds. However, if immigrants achieve their goal of providing their children with increased educational and professional opportunities in the future, the United States will need to continue to allow unauthorized migration or to seek another way to fulfill its lower-end labor needs. Immigrants and their children, whether raised in the United States or in their parents' home communities, are filling a crucial role in the U.S. economy. Although restrictionists might fret about the "costs" of unauthorized immigrants' consumption of public services, a macrolevel perspective reveals that the United States is receiving the labor power of millions of immigrants at a hefty discount, both in wages paid and in the savings from having invested neither in their childhood nor in their care when they retire.[12]

"Anchor Babies"

One of the most virulent manifestations of nationwide anti-immigrant trends is the discourse on "anchor babies," also sometimes referred to as "jackpot babies." Anchor babies are defined by the Federation for American Immigration Reform, a restrictionist organization, as "an offspring of an illegal immigrant or other non-citizen, who under current legal interpretation becomes a United States citizen at birth. These children may instantly qualify for welfare and other state and local benefit programs" (Federation for American Immigration Reform 2009). Within this logic, conniving, contemptible pregnant immigrants cross the border only to "drop" their babies in the emergency rooms of public hospitals, part of a grand plan to take advantage of free emergency medical care and to obtain U.S. citizenship for their children under the protections of the Fourteenth Amendment to the Constitution. The argument follows that immigrants harbor aspirations, but illegitimate ones, designed to strip the United States of costly and limited public resources intended only for citizens. Even though these views sometimes acknowledge that a U.S.-born child can do nothing to affect the immigration status of her parents until reaching the age of twenty-one, when a lengthy sponsorship process can begin, the paranoia and disdain many nativists and restrictionists show toward these alleged anchor babies are pervasive, and they seep into mainstream media coverage and popular discourse surrounding immigration issues. Those who fear this supposed practice of women migrating in order to give birth to babies in the United States seek to amend the Constitution, as discussed in the Epilogue of this book.[13]

I met only one woman out of the many women interviewed in this project who even remotely fit the myth commonly disseminated of undocumented women who migrate in order to give birth to citizens. Articulate and with higher educational attainment than average (she was a college student when she migrated), with plans to return to Mexico as soon as possible, she defies the stereotypes anti-immigrant forces generate. Belén, age twenty, migrated from the city of Cholula, Puebla, in her fifth month of pregnancy. When I asked why, she said, "por los documentos de la nacionalidad" [for citizenship papers]. Her father and five siblings had already migrated to New York, the first thirteen years before. She carefully analyzed the risks and benefits and decided that her baby would have better opportunities as a U.S. citizen, with greater help from the government and educational prospects. She and her husband decided she should migrate first, only a few months after their marriage, before her pregnancy advanced to the point where the crossing would be too risky. She did not have an easy time crossing: she and the other migrants in her group walked three days and nights, then were returned to Mexico by the border patrol. On their second attempt, they walked one full day and were successful in reaching the other side. From there, she rode in a car—she was given preference for the front passenger seat because of her pregnancy—to finally reach New York. Her husband followed shortly thereafter, and when I met her, he was living on Long Island with some of his relatives and working in a flower shop, while she lived in her father's apartment in Brooklyn. They planned to stay a short period, during which her husband would work and save, before returning to Mexico.

Although Belén is the worst nightmare of those restrictionists who spend a great deal of time grumbling about the impact of anchor babies on the nation, she was also a classic immigrant striver. Determined, focused, and educated, she made a rational calculus to choose between options. Ultimately, she made a decision, eminently logical, that her child would be better served having U.S. rather than Mexican citizenship. According to liberal rights perspectives, Belén should be able to bear her child where she chooses. In addition, a strong economic argument can be made that Belén's father and five siblings over more than a decade contributed more to the public coffers with their payment of taxes, and presumably also payroll deductions, to which they may never lay claim, than the several thousand dollars her uncomplicated prenatal care and delivery cost the state of New York. In fact, it could be said that the municipality of Cholula and Belén's family, whose investment in the birth and rearing of six laborers who left the country to dedicate their energy and productivity to the United States economy, are being cheated. They are deprived not only of the affective benefits of the men's presence and family unity but also of the fruits of their labor, including the potential earnings of Belén's child, who is likely to live and work in the United States as an adult.

Exploring some of the experiences of Mexican immigrant women, we can see that even those whose stories confirm restrictionists' worst fears simultaneously defy them. Overall, our understandings should be informed by the complexity of their experiences and the ways that their decision-making processes are constrained by larger political and economic forces at work in their home and host countries as well as in the neocolonial relationship between those countries.

Immigration Law and the Decision to Emigrate

The decisions families make are rendered complicated by the current state of immigration law and migratory flows. Although Mexico and the United States have always had intertwined economies, labor forces, populations, and more, this interdependence and, increasingly, neocolonialist relationship have become increasingly pronounced. The North American Free Trade Agreement (NAFTA) and Mexico's neoliberal economic restructuring have dealt a double blow to many regions of Mexico that previously did not expel migrants.

The region overlapping Puebla, Oaxaca, and Guerrero states, called La Mixteca, from which the majority of Mexican immigrants to New York City hail, did not produce migrant laborers in large numbers until the early 1990s (Lee 2008; Smith 2005). Although NAFTA was touted by its proponents as a means of liberalizing trade between neighbors, it was its understated protectionism that sounded a death knell for the economies of many rural Mexican municipalities. For example, Florida avocado growers lobbied to ensure the market for their crop would be protected from an influx of cheaper Mexican avocados, and thus many Mixteca-region avocado growers who had previously exported vast quantities to the United States ironically no longer could after the signing of the trade agreement (Marroni 2003; Liliana Rivera Sánchez, personal communication, 2002). Moreover, although the Mexican government ensured that caps on the importation of U.S. industrially-grown corn would be in place until 2008, even the limited flows of cheap corn over a decade and a half had a devastating impact.

The inequalities in this area of "free trade" are even more pronounced if we examine the extent to which U.S. corn cultivation is heavily subsidized, while Mexico's corn subsidies were dropped in 1994 in response to pressures for "adjustments" by the United States both during the negotiation over NAFTA and in the bail-out package offered in the wake of the crash of petroleum prices (Farmer 2003, 102–103). These forces converted the traditional home-based *milpa* (small field) corn production from being the backbone of the rural economy to being an idiosyncratic hobby, suitable for retired farmers who do not mind suffering an economic loss in order to savor fresh, homegrown, white-corn tortillas (Hellman 2009). Shockingly, this kind of collateral effect of NAFTA was predicted by the Mexican government, which anticipated that a half million *campesinos*, peasants, would be displaced as a direct result of NAFTA. It was hoped that the rapid industrialization planned to occur both with NAFTA and with neoliberal economic restructuring would enable the transition of these displaced rural people into urban industrial jobs.[14] Small-scale agricultural production became economically unviable as a result of the perfect storm which bombarded Mexico's small-scale agriculturalists: NAFTA, neoliberal restructuration, the peso devaluation in 1994, and a drought that hit the center of the country in the early 1990s. As a result, towns with no history of emigration almost overnight saw their able-bodied youth depart in massive numbers for *el norte.*

On a global scale, the late twentieth and early twenty-first centuries have been characterized by two contradictory trends. On the one hand, globalization has entailed an overspilling of national bounds by trade of capital and goods. Multinational commerce and corporations as well as multilateral trade agreements and economic communities have accelerated transnational economic flows. These trends can also be seen in the political realm: war, attention to refugees, law enforcement, natural-disaster responses, communications, intellectual property, and more are taking on an increasingly international scope. On the other hand, the same time period has witnessed an unprecedented hardening within industrialized nations of the regulations regarding citizenship and residency, limitations on legal migrant flows, attempts to seal borders through militarization, increased stringency in the disbursement of public benefits to noncitizens, and an acceleration of unauthorized migrant flows. In the northern hemisphere, NAFTA has opened up the U.S., Mexican, and Canadian borders to the flows of certain kinds of commerce at the same time that changes in immigration law have been made in attempts to staunch the circulation of people. These regulations have not resulted in a reduction in the number of people who endeavor to migrate to the United States from Mexico and points south, but it has funneled their (illicit) passage through some of the most dangerous and inhospitable sectors of the border.

Ironically, this effort to clamp down cross-border flows has led to longer-term settlement in the United States by unauthorized immigrants. As the border has become more militarized, the crossing more expensive and risky, and opportunities for legal entry less available, families who might once have sent a breadwinner *al norte* on a short-term or seasonal basis have changed their strategies. Many immigrants now opt to stay longer and to relocate the entire family, while single immigrants who in the past might have returned to their hometowns to marry, often opt to settle with a partner and start a family in the United States.

Many immigrants have little desire to stay in the United States for the long term. Many miss their families, their homes, and their communities and wish to return as soon as possible. Most people when asked where they prefer to live, will make elaborate lists of the pros and cons of life in the United States and Mexico. When asked why they have come, as mentioned above, the reasons range from economic need to "para conocer" [to check it out]. When asked why they stay, they also have a variety of reasons: we have yet to save enough money to open the store we are planning; we can't oblige the children to leave, this is their country now; here, the children are being educated in English which will help their future job prospects; or, "ya me acostumbré" [I've become accustomed to it here].[15] One of the problems with the idea of superación is that it is an upward arc with no end in sight. It is rare that someone says, "Me he superado" [I've gotten ahead]. Parents might say, "Here, the children have more opportunities," but they will not usually affirm "We've made it." When the children have grown up in the United States and are unlikely to return "home," families might say, "We've done our part; now it depends on them to take advantage of these opportunities," and thus the torch of superación is passed to the next generation without the trajectory ever ending (see Fernández 2010). Because superación is virtually always sought but rarely achieved, families often remark that they cannot go back: "What do we have to show for ourselves?"

Women in this study told me their various reasons for prolonging or cutting short their stays in the United States. Immigration law increases the stakes in these deliberations, which are not unusual for any family that has embarked on a grand plan. Because so many families cross without authorization, they frequently arrive in the United States already deeply in debt. A coyote might charge Mexicans $900 to $2,000 per person to be smuggled into the country illicitly, more for infants and children.[16] The time it takes to repay this debt and begin to accumulate the capital for a project back home is protracted. Further, as Claudia and her partner calculated, it is sometimes thought prudent to bring the whole family along if the migrant cannot freely visit for the holidays or a funeral without incurring still more debt and the risk of being apprehended. These decisions increase the initial expense of migration and debt load exponentially. When deciding whether to return, if a family has just about enough to accomplish their goals, they might choose to stay on just a little longer to be sure because the risks and expenses associated with return are prohibitive. Others find their goals always recede on the horizon as everyday expenses and needs consume any potential long-term savings; a few choose to cut their losses and return to their home communities, unwilling to expend still more effort and time on their elusive targets. For this reason Massey and Sánchez refer to settlement as a "process more than an event" (2010, 53). Many families who might have wished to be temporary sojourners become reluctant settlers, hunkering down until they achieve their goals or until a chance at legalization makes it possible for them to negotiate their residence, their immigration status, and their ability to move across borders (see Chavez 1988; De Genova 2005; Hellman 2009; Hondagneu-Sotelo 1995; Marcelli and Cornelius 2001; Massey 1986).

Thus, migration occurs in the context of a dependent relationship between the Mexican and U.S. economies, a militarized border, the truncation of economic opportunities in rural Mexico, and the availability of higher-paying jobs in the United States. Finally, migrants' families desire to do what most families wish to do: provide a better life for their children than what they knew. In this particular contextual framework, many of the women in my study embarked on their paths as mothers.

Family Decisions

Determining whether and when to start a family, how many children to have, and whether a mother will enter or remain in the workforce are profoundly private, personal decisions. In addition to the affective motivations to start or to postpone having a family or to enlarge one's family, these considerations have to do with household dynamics, finances, and labor-force participation. They are also influenced in not fully measurable ways by societal trends, technology, and political and economic contexts. In this section, I analyze how these decisions are made by families within a highly fraught political landscape.

Whether and When to Have Children

Many restrictionists imagine that immigrants calculate childbearing in order to maximize their consumption of public benefits. However, data from my study indicate that families find themselves in the United States at a time when it makes sense to them to start a family. This finding is supported by other research, including that reported by Pierette Hondagneu-Sotelo ([2001] 2007) and Sheldon Danziger (cited in Chang 2000).[17] The reasons for these families' presence in the United States are embedded in globalized economics: "Neither America's resources nor its social service system, which is [in] fact one of the stingiest among industrialized nations, is the attraction. The attraction is jobs. . . . The extraction of resources by the United States and other First World nations forces many people in the Third World to migrate to follow their countries' wealth. Moreover the 'draw' of the United States is more accurately described as a calculated pull by the United States and other First World countries on the Third World's most valuable remaining resource: human labor" (Chang 2000, 2–3). Sociologist Hondagneu-Sotelo writes, "Women do not come to the United States to have babies, they have babies here because it is where they live and work" ([2001] 2007, 299). This was true of virtually all the women I interviewed, although I would expand it to say women have babies in the United States because that is where they and their partners live and work.

Contrary to what some might expect, within discourses of superación revealed in my research, the United States is not cast as being self-evidently superior to the rural hometowns from which the majority of interviewees hail. In fact, most women I asked told me they thought that, apart from a few key features, their hometowns offered a better environment for raising children (Smith 2005; Valenzuela 1999). Contrasting New York City with their home community in Mexico, many parents told me that in Mexico children have less danger, less illness, more space, more freedom, more contact with nature, more healthful food, more family ties and support, and more time to use their imaginations, to exercise, and to be with family (see Smith 2005). What children do not have there, many are quick to point out, are educational opportunities and economic security. Although Mexican immigrants frequently consider their country's primary school system to be good, even superior to the schools children attend in New York City, they say youth there have few opportunities to continue their education and that economic concerns often make work a more viable option than study.[18] Many women said that the ability of their spouses and themselves to earn a living and provide for their children without material deprivation, as well as the opportunity to become educated in English, outweighed the positive aspects of life in Mexico. Further, free or subsidized access to medical care is a luxury few say they enjoyed prior to migration (see González 1986, 252). However, these calculations are not easily made, and most families live in a constant state of reassessment. Even to be pregnant and give birth far from their hometowns is an enormous sacrifice for many women and, for some, not one they were happy to make, even while many considered the prenatal care they were able to access in New York City to be superior. Far from scheming to come to the United States to have their babies, families view the decision to start a family in the United States a weighty one, filled with sacrifices and compromises.

Family Size

"See you soon!" The nurse laughed as she discharged Claudia and her new baby from the recovery wing of the labor and delivery ward at Manhattan Hospital. Claudia told me, "She thinks we Mexicans have so many babies that I'll be back here again next year, but not me; I won't be." "Yes, you will, you'll see!" The nurse then turned to me, "They all say the same, and then we see them again in a year." Even while she laughed with the nurse, Claudia shook her head and repeated, "Not me!"

Achieving rapport with health care providers, sharing a laugh, and imagining that if one were to come back again in a year or more that someone would recognize her are aspects of care that patients say they admire at this hospital. Nonetheless, for some providers in this setting, "knowing" their patients means locating them within larger racialized discourses about indigent patients, immigrants, and the "anchor babies" they are imagined to carry. In this dialogue, the nurse implies that she knows this Mexican patient better than she knows herself.

Among prenatal care patients interviewed in this study, decisions about family size had more to do with ideas surrounding the "ideal" number of children than with the availability of contraception, conflicts with partners, traditional Catholic family values, and other factors often associated with fertility. Women and their partners described their efforts to limit the size of their family to the number of children they could raise well, contrasting their views about how many children are ideal with those of their mothers' generation, who they say desired to have as many children as God sent. Virtually all the women interviewed intended to have smaller families than those in which they were raised. Of the sixty-one women for whom I obtained data, the average parity (number of children to whom they had given birth) was 1.1. The women I interviewed were pregnant at the time, and virtually all were of childbearing age, so there is no accurate way of estimating or predicting their life-long fertility. However, when asked, most women said their desired number of children was two or three, averaging out to 2.6. The average number of siblings of the same women was 5.5, while for their spouses the average was 6.0 siblings (see also Sherraden and Barrera 1996). The comments of these women reveal their opinions about family size.

Sandra was raised in a family with six siblings. Pregnant with her first child, she remarked that she wanted to have only two children: "Porque es más fácil se podría decir para mantenerlos, para darles una mejor educación. Ya con muchos niños, no se pueden mantener. Y solo por eso yo pienso que dos están bien" [Because it is easier, one could say, to maintain them, to give them a better education. With too many children, they can't be provided for. And, for that reason alone, I think two is just right].

Brenda was pregnant with her third child. They had planned on two, but she told me, "Nos falló el método" [Our contraceptive method failed]. She grew up in a family with three siblings, and her partner with nine. She did not want as many children as her mother and mother-in-law had: "Más que nada, pues, la atención a los hijos . . . la economía . . . el dinero y crecen . . . y, pues, también para darles lo mejor" [More than anything, well, it's the attention we can give them, finances, money, and they grow . . . and, well, also to be able to give them the best]. She also remarked and was echoed by many women:

> Yo creo que también cuando uno vive en su niñez ciertas cosas, ciertas privacidades [sic], cuando te llegas a ser grande te das cuenta que tener muchos hijos no es . . . conveniente. . . . Sí, y más que nada también la economía, para darles en México . . . por lo mismo, la economía, Usted sabe, está mala. Entonces en mi caso necesitamos, por eso decidimos tener pocos.

> [I also believe that when in one's childhood one has lived with certain things, certain deprivations, when you grow up, you realize that to have many children is not . . . convenient. . . . Yes, and more than anything the economic situation, to be able to provide for them in Mexico, you know, the economy is bad. So, in my case, we're needy, so that's why we decided to have few children.]

In spite of dramatically reduced fertility rates in only a single generation between the women in this study and their mothers' reported childbearing, comments about the assumed excessive fertility of Mexican immigrant women are relatively commonplace.[19] However, they may be rooted in myths about

Mexican families. Residential patterns and family size can be misconstrued. Typically, recent immigrants share an apartment among members of an extended family or multiple, unrelated families. Within these arrangements, a woman who has young children or is pregnant may provide childcare for the other families with whom she resides, thus consolidating and economizing on childcare expenses and responsibilities and allowing the housemates who work to maximize their labor participation.

In general, as seen in the vignette that opened this section, inferences of "excessive" Mexican fertility seem to be routine, even though immigrant families are often determined to have what they consider to be an ideal number of children and usually less than half the number their mothers had.

Mothers in the Workforce: Agency and Subjecthood

Many scholars and activists place a great deal of emphasis on the labor contributions undocumented immigrants make. Sometimes it appears as though immigration reform in its entirety will be determined by the side of the debate that can more convincingly answer a single question: Do undocumented immigrants contribute less than, as much as, or more than they consume? Economists have dedicated countless hours to analyzing consumption of public services, contributions to overall productivity, payroll deductions for Social Security that are never redeemed, and more. They largely agree that immigrants do contribute more than they consume (Griswold 2009; Office of the President 2005; Shierholz 2010; Somerville and Sumption 2009). Further, many immigrants say they pay a sweat equity, and often also income taxes, property taxes, and sales taxes, and ask for little in return. In multiple interviews, people have told me something along the lines of: "We don't take welfare; we contribute to society with our work and our culture." This argument is compelling; however, it presents some hazards for the population that is the focus of this study and reinforces neoliberal models of citizenship that offer only a narrow spectrum of rights in exchange for labor. Sweat-equity arguments for immigrant rights disproportionately valorize immigrants' labor contributions and ignore the (unremunerated, unaccounted for) labor of social reproduction that makes them possible.

Many of the women I interviewed came to the United States to work, having no intention to start a family or to settle in the United States. Some, like Mirna, proudly remark that they take nothing from the government, wishing only to contribute with their labor. For many, their means of coming to the United States and their reasons for staying have more to do with the militarization of the border and the globalization of capital than with any desire they may have had to start a new life in the United States or to settle there for the long term. Further, the United States, with its current neocolonial relationship to its neighbors, extracts the best and most productive years from generations of workers from Latin America and the Caribbean, seeing them return only when they are elderly and infirm.

However, in these discussions activists frequently ignore as inconvenient an almost unspoken reality, but their refusal to discuss it makes them more vulnerable than any other single issue does to attacks by restrictionists. This reality is that many of the women who migrate without authorization to the United States never work a day, or their work history is exceedingly short, truncated for years by pregnancy and childcare responsibilities. This "inconvenient" reality is the Achilles' heel of economic arguments for immigrant rights. How can immigrant activists respond to restrictionists' claims that immigrants consume more than they contribute if some immigrants only consume and are seen, according to short-term quantitative economic measures, to contribute not at all? How can an argument for immigrant rights be built around the stories of women who migrate while pregnant or become pregnant within months of arriving? Close to 90 percent of Mexican immigrant women who gave birth in New York City between 1996 and 2004 were covered by Medicaid (Schwartz and Li, 2002, 2003, 2004; Schwartz, Zimmerman, and Li, 2005, 2006); 58 percent of undocumented women work as opposed to 66 percent of other immigrants and 73 percent of native-born women (Passel and Cohn 2009, 13).[20] Are these statistics that immigrant-rights advocates would do well to bury, or is there value in this information for those who do not hold restrictionist ideologies?

It is necessary to examine the apparent friction between the arguments that many immigrants give for coming to the United States and the realities posed by having a child. A woman who says that she came to better provide for her family and who then becomes pregnant and stops working in the United States poses a contradiction for some, one that cannot simply be swept under the rug for the complications she poses to dominant arguments for immigrant rights. These decisions of women to have children when they do or to become stay-at-home mothers cannot be attributed solely to false consciousness, low levels of education, or lack of access to birth control. Such assumptions are swept up into larger ideologies that have little to do with individual immigrants: views that women might be influenced by their "traditional rural culture" to consider it their destiny to have children, that the use (or not) of contraception is determined solely by men, or that pregnancies are unplanned and a product of conservative Catholic views on abortion and family planning. Some feminist arguments get folded this way, perhaps unwittingly, into strands of population ideologies that view poor women's fertility, "excess" fertility, as a problem to be solved by intervention, education, and "modernization" in general. In this way, women who act in ways that correspond to traditional roles and expectations— follow a partner to the United States, have children, and cease working to care for them—can be viewed within some feminist arguments as insufficiently liberated. Increases in "education" and exposure to the conceptions of female gender roles dominant in industrialized nations are assumed to lead inevitably to fertility decline. Conversations with immigrant women, however, reveal that they are frequently bumping against their family's and neighbors' expectations: defying their mother's notions about family size, defying their mother-in-law's expectations that they will sit passively waiting for a partner's return, defying notions in the United States that only working immigrants are good immigrants— all of this, even while seemingly engaging in "traditional" behaviors: staying at home to bear and care for children.

Most women I interviewed, as will be detailed below, exercised a tremendous amount of agency, seen not only in their decision to migrate but also in their willingness to defy their partners when differences arose about family size, sterilization, and contraception; and most women said that their pregnancies were planned. Far from their fate and curse as women, many of the women described becoming a mother as a dream, a goal, a means to fulfill their own and their family's destiny in ways that are not "traditional" or similar to how they describe their mother's childbearing. Ultimately, having a child is, for many women, a means of superación, not an obstacle to it or detour from it. Further, it offers its own potential for autonomy, a means for creating a personal "web" of interdependence, not completely dominated by affinal kin (Pauli 2008, 173); Rosalind Petchesky advises scholars to be attentive to the "power relations and enabling conditions" within which women articulate and negotiate their claims (1998, 8). Anthropologist Joann Martin describes the "redemptive power of childbirth," noting that "the power of images of women's roles in childbirth and mothering simultaneously subordinated women and provided a model for their entrance into the political arena" (1990, 478, 471). In the context of migration, women told me that having a child can formalize the mutual obligations and ties of a relationship that was previously undefined (see also Dreby 2010). Childbirth and reproduction have been found by scholars to be spheres of female autonomy and power in rural Mexico (Browner and Perdue 1988; Martin 1990).

Further, it is important to notice when decision-making is happening at the level of the family, not simply the individual. A woman's labor-force participation or lack thereof cannot be interpreted entirely through examination of her life as an individual. Instead, we must consider the family as a political subject in which individuals play roles that are complementary to and not reducible to the roles other members play (Pallares 2009). Interestingly, in their study of compliance with medical mandates during pregnancy, Carole Browner and Nancy Press found that only Latina women named "cultural" reasons for defying a doctor's orders (1996, 151)—for example, feeling pressure to eat something during a family meal that their obstetrician had told them to avoid. Although it seems likely Latinas are not the only women to receive family pressure while pregnant, it is notable that some may view the family's perspectives as more mandatory than a doctor's advice.

Although such a view poses challenges to some feminist arguments about women's autonomy, it offers an alternative way to look at the decision by some women to migrate while pregnant or to become pregnant shortly after arrival. Of course, measuring women's ability to act as agents in their own lives is not as simple as examining their empowered or subjugated interactions with the biomedical establishment, patriarchal social norms, or their own family members and partners. Browner has found "women are neither agents acting solely on their free will or completely constrained by the actions of men" (2000, 784; also Martin 1990, 471), an echoing of Karl Marx's maxim that "men make their own history, but they do not make it as they please" ([1852] 2008, 15). Constraints are also imposed on women's agency by the larger structural forces that prompted their migration to the United States and insertion into public health care facilities in New York. Julia Pauli writes, "Female agency is shaped not only by the male partner's interests, support, or nonsupport" but has "relational dimensions" (2008, 172). Agency is a necessary premise of citizenship: "Autonomy and consciousness are attributes of the presumed unique, creative individuality of modern subjects, but also of their dialogical engagement with fellow citizens" (Yuval-Davis and Werbner 1999, 12).

Political scientist Amalia Pallares theorizes the importance of viewing the family as a political subject (2009, 2010). This idea, in conjunction with discourses of superación, offers a fruitful means for interpreting the decisions made about where and when to have children and how many to have. If the family is viewed as a political subject, the state is, of necessity, required to contend with families as pluralities, not as individuals who may or may not hold citizenship rights. This requirement is also a corrective to what has been described as "a long historical legacy of people of color being incorporated into the United States through coercive systems of labor that do not recognize family rights" (Hondagneu-Sotelo and Avila 1997, 568). A family's goal of superación may, indeed, be served well by a mother who stays at home to bear and raise children while her spouse works, and it is our task as scholars of immigration to explore and explain why that is the case, not simply to pretend she does not exist. Deeper attention to the political subjecthood of immigrant mothers offers new ways to conceptualize citizenship.

Focusing on the family as a political subject does not offer a solution to basic issues of women's empowerment and equality. Some women in this study described being beaten, manipulated, coerced, and ordered around by their partners, natal kin, affinal kin, employers, smugglers, and even house-mates. To look at families as a relevant unit of social analysis, a site for decision-making, resource allocation, emotional and economic support, and more does not mean that inequalities within families can be overlooked. It offers, however, an important corrective to the classical liberal (and now neoliberal) conceptions of the individual subject as the repository and both the beginning and end points of rights.

Within changing conceptualizations of marriage, romance, decision-making, family size, child-rearing, and more, women and men articulate their ideal relationship, and the family lives in conversation with and contradistinction to those of their partners, parents, neighbors, and siblings. They also contend with lasting structural and social relationships, habits, and tendencies with which they were raised as well as economic needs that often thwart their abilities to realize their ideal, modern lives (Dreby 2010; Gutmann 1996; Hirsch 2003; Islas 2010; Napolitano 2002). To categorize the relatively low rates of workforce participation among undocumented women immigrants compared with male immigrants and female nonimmigrants (Passel 2005) as a remnant of less than modern patriarchal social norms under which women are supposed to be home, pregnant, and child-rearing is to ignore the strategic and empowered decisions women and their family members make to reunite their families, begin families after migration, enter or leave the workforce, or engage in full-time childcare in complex circumstances (Dreby 2010; Gutierrez 2008; Hondagneu-Sotelo [2001] 2007, 299).

The remaining chapters in this book tell this story, which is not a simple one. For many women, migrating to the United States and having a baby in a hospital, even if that implies a rupture from female kin networks and other support back home, is a sign of having made progress in their project of superación. Many women were proud to have their babies at the public hospital in which I conducted my research, and they frequently felt that with their baby's birth they were already on track to improving his or her life chances. Having a baby does not diminish families' efforts at superación; on the contrary it is some-times an important marker along their path toward it. And childbearing and child-rearing are not unproductive within strictly economic views. We need to examine how it is that the earnest, eager strivings of immigrant families to make a new start, get ahead, and do what is best for their families get twisted both by anti-immigrant ideologies surrounding anchor babies and consumption of public resources and also by public health providers whose protocols of care do not allow room for aspiration. This is a story I continue to tell in the following chapters.

Chapter 3

Remembering Reproductive Care in Rural Mexico

Luisa was busy. Even while she chatted amiably, she diligently worked, writing onto the sketch of her family tree the names, birth dates, and birth weights of all of the many grandchildren given her by her seven children. Over several weeks, I had conducted participant observation with a women's group at the Queens community center of a large immigrant-rights organization. Once per week a mixed-age group of Mexican women gathered, some with their babies, some with toddlers and preschoolers who played with crayons, blocks, or puzzles while we talked. For three weeks, a visiting Mexican psychologist had run a workshop on self-esteem and prevention of domestic violence. When it finished, the director of the center, María Zúñiga, and I came up with the idea of doing a project on family trees.

Part art project, part community-building activity, and in part to further my research, the family trees were eagerly begun. Over one morning's session, we sketched kinship charts on plain paper. Although kinship charts are a time-honored anthropological tradition used by researchers to map local ideas of relatedness, residence and marriage patterns, and more, I was not trained in graduate school to make them or even how to read them, although one of my professors warned us he was once quizzed on them during a job interview. Family trees are essentially the same practice, but they are used by nonspecialists to map their own genealogies. I told the women the little I knew about methods of notation: a circle for a woman, a triangle for a man, a horizontal bar for a marriage, vertical lines to connect children to their parents' union, age order indicated from left to right, and so on. I soon found my knowledge tapped out when I was asked how to render adoptive children and the unusual family

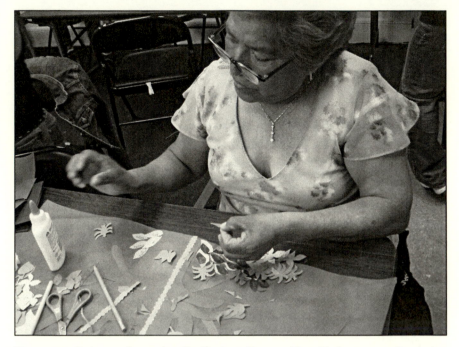

Figure 1 Luisa works on her family tree, Queens, New York, community center, May 2007. Photo by the author.

pattern of two sisters who had married a pair of brothers, thus intertwining their lineages. I encouraged everyone to use horizontal rows for each generation, attaching additional sheets of paper as necessary to render their family trees. Many women struggled with squeezing in everyone. These women's reckoning of their families involved a great deal of horizontal space—many children in each generation—and the family trees usually went back only as far as grandparents or, in some cases, great-grandparents. I also realized that kinship charts are inadequate when it comes to representing one's spouse's family, about whom many of the women knew a great deal and whom they considered critical to any rendering of their family.

When we began transferring the kinship charts to a large family tree made of a brown paper trunk placed on a red paper background, with leaves for each member of the family, the women discussed their families. Marta and Isabel, sisters, had struggled making their kinship charts, wondering how to represent the intertwining of their natal family and that of their husbands, who are brothers. To represent their families, they found it necessary to have the same individual appear twice—both sister and *concuña*.[1] But when offered the fluid format of an image of a tree, they represented their unique family beautifully by having branches of two trees intertwine in space without it being necessary to repeat the same individuals. Luisa cut out dozens of multi-colored leaves in multiple shapes—some representing entire families. She used colors as well as shapes symbolically, giving one leaf to each of her own children and grandchildren but assigning her aunts' and uncles' offspring a single leaf with four, five, seven sections, as necessary, to indicate each of their children. She had a pile of fallen leaves to the left of her tree, symbolizing all of the dead.

Luisa is unusual; there are not many Mexican grandmothers in New York. Only 1.7 percent of the Mexican population of New York City is over 62 years of age, while the median age is 25.7 years (U.S. Census Bureau 2006, 2007, 2008). Luisa was highly critical of younger Mexican women living in New York City, who she felt exhibited less fortitude than her generation had. During the family-tree activity, she took the opportunity to explain to me and to the half dozen other younger women at the table the ways she found her compatriots today to be less resilient than she was. She raised her seven children in rural Puebla state. All but the seventh were born at home with a *partera*, a lay mid-wife, without complications, she said. The last, who she said weighed ten and half pounds, was born in a clinic by caesarean section.

In her view, mothers in the United States had it too easy, referring to her countrywomen. She said mockingly that women in the United States have everything paid for by the state; they receive welfare and everything is free. And yet they complain, "'Ay, tengo que ir a lavar,' y eso que van a la esquina a la lavandería y pagan, y nada más. Yo iba con mis siete niños al río a lavar, y tomaba todo el dia en ir, lavar, y después volver, horas caminando" ['Ay, I have to do laundry,' even though they just have to go to the corner, pay, and that's that! I had to take my seven children to the river to wash. It took all day to get there, wash, and come home, hours of walking]. She said that she would tie her youngest to her belly with a hammock for the journey, and when she arrived at the riverside she tied the hammock in a tree. She said she invented a means of attaching a nipple to a sack so the baby could feed himself. Proudly, she recounted that he never choked, lost the nipple, spilled the milk, or cried. Her children helped her and never complained. She said she could make four eggs feed the whole family, while in the United States each member of the family wants two eggs apiece. She said women in the United States have no responsi-bilities and complain more; when they are pregnant they hold their backs and say, "¡Ay, mi cintura!, ¡Ay, mi espalda!" [Ay, my waist! Ay, my back!]. She said her children never had any problems, but in New York City almost every child is in speech therapy, needs asthma medication, sees a doctor every week. Luisa described her role as a mother of young children as being one of work, and her children, for their part, could not trouble her by having problems or individual needs. In this way, she could handle all seven of them, and she implied that a woman of this generation would never be able to do that.

The younger women had listened to Luisa silently, but then Isabel interrupted and said that it is not that children have more illness in the United States but rather a mother can take the time to spend with a child, to really focus on the child's needs. One has fewer children, and there are more services if a child needs them. In Mexico, she said, her son could not have speech therapy every day; if he did not speak, there would not be any services for him. She said that immigrant women have fewer children and focus on them; they raise them well.

I asked Luisa whether she thought women suffered more in pregnancy in the United States. She said yes; she never had any problems in her seven pregnancies. Luisa expresses here a strand of the arguments made to explain why pregnancy and childbirth are so different in Mexico and the United States. Many women, especially older women like Luisa who had children prior to migrating, feel that their compatriots are constitutionally altered by their migration. This change is thought to occur in many ways. Some say it is attributable to the diet that migrants consume in the United States. *Comida chatarra*, junk food, makes them weaker, more prone to illness than the farm-to-table fare to which they were accustomed *en el pueblo.*[2] As one woman said, "Una mexicana se cuida mejor, salen gorditos y sanos los bebés. Es por la alimentación" [A Mexican takes better care of herself. The babies come out fat and healthy. It's because of the diet]. Others say that life in New York is more "comfortable": living in an apartment in which heat, hot water, and laundry facilities are frequently available and in which obtaining food requires a quick jaunt to the supermarket makes women "soft." Further, Luisa implies, by being relieved of the extreme physical demands of living in a rural environment, where caring for animals, a garden, sometimes a milpa of corn, without the appliances that make laundry, for example, easy, women in New York become lazy and weak. These women complain about their pregnancies in ways that women like Luisa claim they never had the time or inclination to do.

In these arguments, a medical approach to pregnancy, conceived of as a pathology requiring specific medical interventions and care, becomes necessary.[3] Women who migrate, in Luisa's estimation, simply are not capable of having the kind of uncomplicated pregnancy that she had and thus require a different kind of prenatal care. Similarly, Matthew Gutmann found in his research in rural Oaxaca that the United States was construed by some traditional healers as "an especially noxious source of illness" (2007, 183). Jacqueline, similarly, told me that pregnancy is safer in Mexico; in New York, there are more complications and "más sindromes" [more syndromes], and, accordingly, "más atención." She told me about a midwife who lived around the corner from her in Cholula; this woman delivered scores of babies and only rarely dealt with any complications requiring a hospital transfer. She told me the midwife never studied but just had a lot of experience, making a gesture indicating her wonder that someone could have such good results without training.

The interchange between Luisa and Isabel follows rather predictable lines: an elder complains about the younger generation, who, in her view, would not have survived a day in her shoes, while younger women become irritated and point out that they have different priorities, concerns, and worries than their mothers had back *en el rancho,* as people sometimes call their rural hamlets (Raison 2007). Also described here are the contours of ideas not only about changing times but also about changing places, values, and aspirations. Although personhood for women in rural Mexico historically centers on motherhood and all the abnegation and suffering that it is thought to entail, modern personhood rests on notions of the empowered individual (Napolitano 2002, 166). Mexican immigrant women are told by their mothers that becoming a woman involves endurance and sacrifice as well as devotion to children but envision for themselves a life based on companionship, friendship, and independence (Hirsch 2003; Napolitano 2002; Pauli 2008). Isabel and others among the younger mothers in the group frequently described the challenges they faced in budgeting their family's expenses, obtaining health care, advocating for their children in public schools, working part or full time to make ends meet, and more. They argued that back *en el pueblo* the family and the land provided everything: there was no need to pay rent or utilities, the schools did not expect such a high level of parental involvement or advocacy, and children were expected simply to obey, not to develop as individuals.

In one of these sessions, I brought up my concerns that my nearly two-year-old child was not yet talking much. Isabel had already told me that her son was receiving almost daily speech therapy. She told me about her experiences of having him evaluated and obtaining state-subsidized services under New York State's Early Intervention Program. Luisa had different advice: she told me to take a key, wash it with soap and water, go to church to have the key blessed, and then put it into my son's mouth to "unlock" his tongue. She recounted the many times she had seen late talkers cured by this *remedio casero,* home remedy. Isabel, who felt speech therapy was helping her son, eagerly said that she would try the trick with the key: "It can't hurt!" she exclaimed.

Sources of Information about Pregnancy and Childbirth in Rural Mexico

Although it must be a nearly universal experience that young mothers alternately embrace and bristle at the advice of their mothers and mothers-in-law and generational friction is at least partly to blame for pendulum swings in parenting styles, in the interactions I have described there is a more complex dynamic. Women like Isabel and Luisa not only must bridge a generational divide when comparing their experiences as mothers but must also contend with the vast distance created by migration, in which few of the day-to-day activities Luisa associates with mothering are the same for Isabel. At the same time, their hometowns have been transformed too, so that even Luisa's daughters who continue to live in her pueblo do not walk for hours to the river to do laundry. The landscape of pregnancy, childbirth, and child-rearing practices has been transformed in rural communities in Mexico in ways that neither Isabel nor Luisa may fully appreciate. Having migrated, they are likely to compress the notions of *here* and *there* with those of *now* and *then*. As such, many women, like Isabel, who have given birth to their children in the United States contrast their experiences with those of their mothers without always acknowledging that, had they stayed in Mexico to start a family, they likely would have experienced childbirth and pregnancy differently than their own mothers did.

I trace this disconnect of space and time in this chapter, listening to what women say about pregnancy and childbirth "back" in Mexico in order to trace how their ideas about the ways their mothers managed these life events affect their own dispositions as mothers. By talking also to women who are prenatal care providers, mothers, and grandmothers in some of the parts of Mexico where the migrants in New York were born, I have found that change occurs in all places at once. Change does not occur only for those who migrate, and in the distance between change that is noticed and commented on and change that is not important attitudes about mothering and care practices during pregnancy and childbirth are revealed.

The attitudes women have toward pregnancy and childbirth in their hometowns have everything to do with their views of their mothers' and grandmothers' lives and of their own childhood. Women who have migrated may feel nostalgia toward many aspects of life "back home," but they also sometimes bid good riddance to those aspects of life in rural Mexico that they associate with the truncation of opportunity, poverty, and, in some cases, gender violence, the aspects of rural life that drove them to migrate. Gutmann writes about the views of residents of Santo Domingo, a working-class, former squatter settlement in Mexico City, toward rural life: "One factor involved in the disparaging remarks about the campo from residents of Santo Domingo who come from rural areas is that these people are often remembering less-than-contented childhoods. This means both that unhappiness in childhood may act as a filter on their memories, and more significantly, that despite periodic return visits to see family in the campo, they are most familiar with their natal villages of fifteen or twenty years ago, and even before that" (1996, 63).[4]

This issue of familiarity is also of heightened relevance to the women who participated in this study. Although the people Gutmann interviewed in Mexico City had access to their natal villages fettered only, perhaps, by economic means, time, and desire to travel, the women I interviewed in New York City, mostly undocumented immigrants, were largely unable to travel back to Mexico. Although return travel is relatively simple and inexpensive, reentry to the United States with the current militarized border is prohibitively expensive and dangerous (Massey and Sánchez 2010). Thus, like residents of Santo Domingo, they, too, are most familiar with their natal villages of years before, but that familiarity has not been refreshed except through reports from relatives who phone, e-mail, send videos, and migrate or travel to the United States. As such, their opinions and knowledge about life *en el rancho* are shaped in powerful and yet unpredictable ways by emotional factors such as nostalgia, bitterness, resentment, homesickness, and loss, all heightened by protracted separations of space and time.

For this reason, I attend to the narration of changing practices of care during pregnancy and childbirth in the hometowns from which the women I interviewed hail. A vast amount of anthropological work has examined reproductive care practices in the same parts of Mexico in which I briefly conducted research. I make little reference to that work here, not because it is not important and valid scholarship—it is. But my purpose here is not to provide a survey of pregnancy and birth practices but rather to trace discourses surrounding those practices and the circulation of those discourses among Mexican immigrants in New York City. What are the elements of traditional practices that women comment on as they sit in a New York City prenatal clinic? Which features that they associate with birth in their hometown in Mexico do they miss and which do they feel privileged to have left behind? How do their attitudes about what they perceive to be the norms surrounding pregnancy and childbirth affect their disposition toward the prenatal care they receive in New York City?

How and why does migration sometimes produce a spatial and a temporal dissonance between here and now, there and then?

I describe here interviews with two parteras, as well as a botanist and family members of migrant women in Puebla and Oaxaca states. In Oaxaca City, I interviewed Violeta, a *partera empírica*, an "empirical" midwife, who is no longer actively practicing but who delivered scores of babies in her natal village, Santa María Zoohochí, as well as in Río Blanco, the working-class neighborhood in Oaxaca City to which she migrated decades earlier. I interviewed her at her home with her daughter, a medical doctor in general practice. In the town of Ixtlán de Juárez, in the Sierra de Juárez, northeastern Oaxaca state, I interviewed Prudencia, a midwife who practices in the state-funded center for natural health in that town, adjacent to a public health clinic. She also practices in her hometown, San Pedro de Yaneri. In addition, I discussed herbal remedies and properties of plants with a botanist at the Jardín Botánico Elia Bravo Hollis, near Zapotitlán Salinas, Puebla state, and birth practices with practicing anthropologists living in Oaxaca. I spent time there with family members of New York City–dwelling migrants, especially the family of María Pacheco, whose experiences are described at length in this book.

The Role of Mothers-in-Law

Historically in most regions of Mexico, families followed a virilocal residence pattern (Gutmann 1996, 166; Pauli 2008). Anthropological kinship and residence terms are infrequently used in anthropology today, in keeping, perhaps, with the ways that contemporary urban social life has ruptured many of the traditional patterns for forming a family.[5] However, in some of the rural areas of Puebla, Oaxaca, and Guerrero states, also known as La Mixteca, virilocal residence continues to be the most common pattern, and even when it is not adhered to, this pattern is described as the norm on which other arrangements are variations. An analysis of how such patterns can mold social life is relevant. Virilocal residence means that when couples embark on their lives together, they do so in the young man's parents' home. This practice contributes to what Judith Adler Hellman has called "the tyranny of the mother-in-law" (2009), and Julia Pauli has called "the mother-in-law system" (2008, 182). In Hellman's research, many informants named their desire for freedom from such a residential arrangement as a major factor both in their initial decision to migrate as well as in their ongoing resolve to stay on in the United States (2009; also Pauli 2008; Stephen 1991).

In interviews, many women spoke about friction and problems with their *suegra*, mother-in-law. One of the most unforgivable actions of a mother-in-law seemed to be not defending her daughter-in-law from abuse or even instigating it. However, at the same time, many women considered distance from this kind of residence pattern to be a significant hardship. Although some women said their mother-in-law could not or would not care for them the way their own mother might have, ties to a web of female kin, whether affinal or consanguine, is one of the aspects of life in Mexico that immigrant women miss most during pregnancy and the postpartum period in the United States. In a virilocal residence pattern, frequently the birth of a child consecrates the couple's relationship and legitimizes it in the view of relatives and neighbors. Although the suegra may or may not have fondness or respect for her daughter-in-law, she typically has a deep interest in protecting and nurturing—from conception forward—her future grandchild, who in important ways belongs to her.

One mother, Josefina, described how a mother-in-law can be possessive about her grandchildren. Josefina's husband, Juan, was born in Mexico but had grown up in the Bronx. When he reached young adulthood, he went back to his parents' hometown and there met Josefina. Following a period of courtship, they decided to start a family together, and she became pregnant. When she was due to deliver, she was advised by her medical provider that she would require a cesarean section. Unable to obtain resources for such a procedure, Juan phoned his mother in the Bronx, who worked cleaning private homes in Manhattan. Josefina's mother-in-law sent the money for the surgery. A few months later, she phoned the couple and told them she wanted the child brought to her. Appalled and unwilling to part with her child, Josefina decided to migrate to the United States with the baby. The baby was sent on an airplane with someone who had documents to travel, while Josefina hired a coyote (incurring further debts to her mother-in-law) and arrived in the Bronx a short time later.[6] Juan followed soon after, under pressure from his wife and mother to work as much as he could to pay back these debts. While living in the Bronx, Josefina was regularly told by her mother-in-law that if she displeased her, she would be sent back, but the child would remain: the mother-in-law considered the child hers because she had paid for him, she said. Eventually, the mother-in-law's possessiveness led the couple to find another apartment, but Josefina cried to me that she still felt suffocated by the woman's demands. I asked her if Juan's mother behaved the same way toward their younger son, a baby who was born about a year after Josefina's arrival in New York; she said no; that child had been born in a public hospital, free of charge; Josefina did not need to defend her rights over him. On the contrary, Josefina sometimes struggled to get her mother-in-law to "tomarlo en cuenta al bebé" [take the baby into consideration] because the woman paid more attention to her elder grandson.

Regardless of the possibility of problems with in-laws, within notions of pregnancy described for rural Mexico by study participants, the pregnant mother and all her relatives have a tremendous role to play in ensuring the health of the pregnancy and producing a healthy child. Pregnancy advice, *consejos*, issued by female kin and many others, is intended not only as a guide but as a mandate for the pregnant mother: this advice is simple, straightforward, easy to remember, and is considered absolutely essential to the wellbeing of the mother and baby.

Pregnancy Care Practices

Anthropologist Tsipy Ivry writes about how pregnancy is conceived differently in distinct cultural settings: each culture has its own "paradigms of thinking about persons, and how they come into being, that go beyond biomedicine" (2010, 11). In Israel, she writes, nutrition, the mother's attitude toward her pregnancy, her investment in strategies to nurture or care for herself or her fetus are considered irrelevant to the outcome of the pregnancy, which is viewed largely to be genetically determined. In contrast, in Japan, she found that it is considered a woman's responsibility to produce a healthy fetus, a project involving not only nutritional mandates but the expectation that the womb will be kept warm, the baby in utero spoken with and "cheered up," and more. Although the present study is not about Mexican theories surrounding pregnancy generally, my research does support the assertion that Mexican families consider themselves to be responsible for healthy pregnancies and childbirths (Sesia 1996). That participants in this study located responsibility for care of their pregnancies and the pregnant mother among all members of the family indicates that this responsibility is viewed as too much for the mother to handle alone. Indeed, rallying around care for the pregnant woman was described in ways that indicate that it produces a significant amount of joy and bonding among family members. Families engage in many different strategies and practices to care for the pregnant woman and ensure her and her baby's health.

Nevertheless, women in this study placed a far greater emphasis on care practices for the laboring and postpartum mother and child than on gestation. The care practices that are associated with pregnancy are remarkably simple; the advice most women describe receiving is reducible to a few mandates: eat well, walk a lot, and do not carry heavy things. Even though some prenatal care practices, such as indulgence of *antojos,* cravings, and *sobada,* massage, are quite elaborate, birth and the forty-day period that follows are subject to a greater complexity of practices by specialists who tend to mother and child with a wealth of foods, herbs, and devices (Sesia 1996). Women in this study did not explicitly remark on pregnancy as being less susceptible to intervention than childbirth and the postpartum period. However, if, following Ivry, the practices and attitudes associated with gestation are examined, we may locate certain "etiologies of fetal [and maternal] health and illness" (2010, 233). It is an assertion of this book that one of the "advantages" or "protective features" contributing to the health of Mexican immigrant women and their babies during pregnancy and childbirth is the view that reproduction is a blessing and an endeavor that women are uniquely capable—even destined—to accomplish. For many women, pregnancy is not an illness that is inherently dangerous in normal circumstances; it does not even require supervision by specialists, although certain complications and labor do. Anthropologist Paola Sesia, writing about research with lay midwives in the Isthmus of Tehuantepec in Oaxaca state in the early to mid-1990s, wrote, "The notion of 'risk' is a biomedical one, mostly unknown to local midwives" (1996, 130).

For this reason, in discussing theories about pregnancy among women who live in or who have migrated from rural Mexico, it is possible we might even choose to discard Ivry's phrasing in that *etiologies* refers to origins of an illness or disease. Maternal health and illness have not necessarily been considered together in many rural Mexican contexts historically, although with the increased diffusion of biomedical models of obstetric care, "risk" is certainly more commonly discussed today than it was in the past. When women describe caring for themselves and obtaining care from others during pregnancy, they do not necessarily do so within a framework of implicit risk, and, in fact, the rise of discourses of risk may be a measure of the impact both of immigration and of the Mexican government's expansion of biomedical public health care to rural communities.

Let's examine some of the features that women describe when talking about "typical" pregnancy experiences in their hometowns, as well as the kinds of food and home remedies they consume. The story of Marisol, which opened this book, describes a typical dynamic of care during pregnancy. Marisol's mother-in-law made her chicken soup when she was nauseated. Other women describe being given tea and warm tortillas. When Claudia was sick, her mother recommended that she drink hot water with lemon. Her mother-in-law, unlike her own mother, enjoyed eating meat at every meal, while Claudia was accustomed to a more vegetable-based diet. She was never quite comfortable living in her in-laws' home and was pleased that after immigrating she could make her own decisions about what to cook and eat. Nevertheless, her mother-in-law took her obligation to care for Claudia seriously and made sure to express to her son the importance of indulging his wife's cravings, *consentirle sus antojos.*

Consentir antojos is one of the most commonly mentioned ways that family members become directly involved in a pregnant woman's diet. Although a pregnant woman's cravings have taken on the level of caricature in the United States, with images of pregnant women sending their husbands on midnight runs for pickles and ice cream, in Mexico, interviewees told me, cravings must be indulged. As strange as they may seem, they are viewed as a sign that the body needs something in particular.[7] Lila and Brenda described an overwhelming need to eat dirt during their pregnancies. This is not an uncommon occurrence: obstetrical literature calls it pica, a craving for nonfood substances such as soil or chalk (Rothenberg, Manalo, and Jiang 1999; Simpson et al. 1994). Lila said she was so consumed with that desire that she convinced a local brick mason to give her a brick to eat: "Oiga no sea malito, regáleme un ladrillo para un cafecito. . . . Es que, como que se hacía que estaba crudo y lo partía y se desmoronaba bien rico y sí, ese fue mi antojo" [Hey, don't be mean, give me a little brick to make a cup of coffee. . . . It's just that as he was working with it, it looked like it was raw, and it split and crumbled in a really delicious way, and that was my craving]. She tells the brick mason not to be "mean": that to deny her what she was craving, as strange as it was, would be cruel. In her recounting of the episode, she used diminutives (*malito, cafecito*) associated with affectionate or supplicating interactions, and she used *regáleme*, a verb for giving a gift.[8]

In this way, the discursive construction of antojos and the ways women talk about them show how claims are indulged, even in circumstances of scarcity or, in this case, oddity. Most cravings are for rather more edible items: fruit, sometimes sprinkled with powdered dry chile, lemon, and salt; tamarind or quince sweets; *licuados* (smoothies); cake; or *pan dulce* (sweet bread). Favorably contrasting their experiences after migrating to New York with their lives before, many women said they became able to fulfill their cravings in ways that they were unable to during pregnancies in Mexico. In their mother-in-law's house, to avoid being a burden or because of scant resources, women described having to quiet their cravings. They feared, however, that they were possibly denying their baby needed nutrients. Lorena said that when she was pregnant in Mexico, she did not experience cravings. "No me antojaba porque sabía que no se podía" [I did not have cravings because I knew I couldn't]. In her fourth pregnancy, in New York, in contrast, she said, "Ahora, sí, una sandía, McDonald's, comida china" [Now, yes, watermelon, McDonald's, Chinese food]. In this way, she contradicts characterizations of cravings as indexical of a nutritional deficiency and out of women's conscious control, noting she was able to manipulate her cravings, staving them off because of the

scarcity of resources to fulfill them. She told me that a failure to indulge cravings could result in a miscarriage and cause suffering to the pregnant mother,
but, luckily, she avoided having them in her early pregnancies.

Care Specialists and the Use of Herbal Remedies

In parts of rural Mexico, historically, a range of specialists have focused on
reproductive needs: conception, gestation, labor, and recovery. These specialists go by various names, some of which are used interchangeably and others
precisely; some refer only to women and others seem most often to be used in
reference to men. The terms include *parteras, brujos, bañeras, yerberos, hueseros,* and *sobadores*; sometimes they are glossed under the heading *curandero,*
healer. Later, we will see how some of the knowledge of these specialists is
accessible to immigrant women in New York. In Nahuatl, in the pre-Colombian
epoch, parteras were called *temixhihuatiani,* and their expertise was said to
derive at least in part from their gender: "Sólo una mujer puede cuidar a otra
mujer, pues sólo ella es capaz de entender los trances por los que atraviesa otra
mujer" [Only a woman can care for another woman because only she is capable
of understanding the difficult moments a woman goes through] (Ramírez
Carillo 2001, 1; see Alatorre Wynter 1994). A brujo, a male "witch" or healer,
may specialize in a variety of healing arts and magic. Bañeras may be appren-
tices to parteras, although sometimes their expertise is considered complementary and parallel to that of parteras. Bañeras specialize in the use of steam and
dry heat along with herbs in special baths referred to as *temazcales* or, in the
absence of a temazcal, at home (see Gutmann 2007, 175). Yerberos specialize in
the use of medicinal plants, *hierbas.* Sobadores are experts in deep-tissue massage who can turn a fetus that is breech, promote conception, cure muscle
aches, and treat kidney problems. Hueseros do bone and joint work to set bro-
ken bones and more. Historically, a range of these specialists would practice in
any sizable rural community, but today the few that remain sometimes cover
wide swaths of territory or do double duty. It seems that some parteras do the
work of bañeras, and they will also offer sobadas to their clients. Brujos and
sobadores, likewise, are sometimes one and the same.

In Mexico, although the insertion of the federal health system into rural
towns has often correlated negatively with the prevalence of traditional medicine, this knowledge has also been subject to various official and grassroots
efforts to preserve it. Federal funding is inconsistent and fickle, but there are
notable efforts. For example, in Puebla state, the botanical garden Jardín
Botánico Elia Bravo Hollis, near Zapotitlán Salinas, is dedicated to preserving
native plants as well as the knowledge of their use. In Tlaxiaco, Oaxaca, an

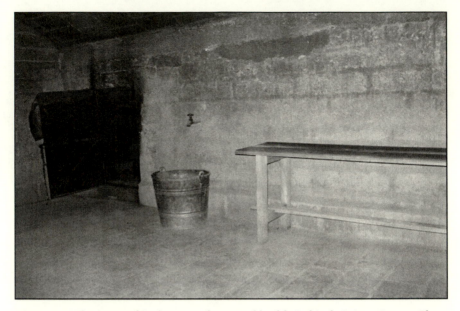

Figure 2   The temazcal in the center for natural health, Ixtlán de Juárez, Oaxaca. Photo by the author.

organization founded in the mid-1980s by traditional healers called the Organización de Médicos Indígenas de la Mixteca works to conserve and promote indigenous medicine, including the use of plants, animals, minerals, and waters for healing. Previously funded by the Instituto Nacional Indigenista, the organization no longer receives federal funding, and although in 2005 it had several health centers, botanical gardens, and pharmacies, it seems now to be on the decline (Organización de Médicos Indígenas de la Mixteca 2009). Many Mexican universities also have programs in ethnobotany and related fields, which are dedicated to preserving knowledge about plants as well as to providing training programs for midwives and other practitioners of "indigenous medicine," and foreign biologists are a frequent sight in Mexico.[9]

In addition to specialists, many lay people boast of a rich knowledge of traditional medicine. Many research participants remarked on what they perceived to be the overuse in the United States of pharmaceuticals for common illnesses and pain, in contrast to the use of herbal remedies, which they were accustomed to in Mexico. Many women who enthusiastically embraced a biomedical approach to pregnancy nevertheless said they would not use over-the-counter pain relievers or cold medicine during pregnancy, even if their providers suggested it. As we will see later, they also generally expressed a disinclination toward use of chemical pain relief during labor and delivery.

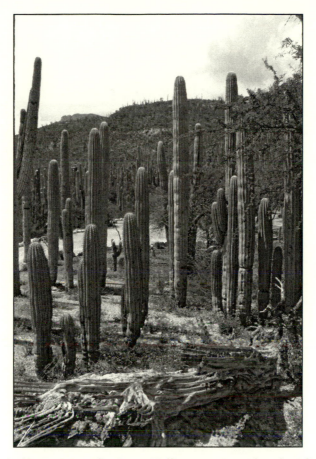

Figure 3   Jardín Botánico Elia Bravo Hollis, near Zapotitlán de Salinas, Puebla. Photo by the author.

The midwives I interviewed in Oaxaca described many plants and herbs used for a variety of purposes prior to conception, during gestation, during labor, and following childbirth.[10] *Ruda* (*Ruta graveolens*) is used for many purposes. It can be an abortifacient, but also can be used in small quantities to treat nausea in the first trimester. *Hierba maestra* (*Artemisia absinthium linnaeus*) is used as well. *Manzanilla*, chamomile, is used for stomach upsets, anxiety, and constipation. *Cedro* (*Cedrela odorata*) is used in a tea to produce milk and restore the uterus. *Té de canela,* cinnamon tea, is avoided during the first trimester as it can cause miscarriage but may be used to induce labor at the end of pregnancy.

Although most women I interviewed in New York mentioned the use of herbs and other remedios caseros during pregnancy, many of them struggled to remember the names or proportions of the plants used. María Pacheco told me that her mother sent packets of herbs with a cousin, with instructions for their use. As we will see in the next chapter, her husband prepared the herbs for her, but neither of them knew the precise names for them. Other women told me they were able to procure some of the herbs at Mexican stores in New York, including *papalo* (*Porophyllum ruderale*), which is a green-leafed herb eaten with the fresh stems of *pepichas* (*Porophyllum tagetoides*); it is made into salsas or cooked in stews. *Te-quesquite*, a mineral salt, was mentioned as a remedy taken in water. For headaches and body aches, massage with alcohol or eucalyptus were discussed.

Belén, age twenty, was one of the few women I interviewed in New York who could confidently name several of the herbs used in Mexico in homeopathic remedies during pregnancy and postpartum, including *pirul* (*Schinus molle*), *alcanfor* (*Cinnamomum camphora*), *romero* (*Rosmarinus officinalis*), *laurel* (*Lauraceae*), and *chichicastle* (*Urtica chamaedryoides*).[11] She also named a mix of sulfur and egg as a treatment. In spite of her knowledge of home remedies, Belén attributed their use to a lack of satisfactory alternatives.

Birth and Postpartum Practices

When I asked Mexican immigrant women about childbirth in their hometowns, many started off by highlighting the ways it negatively compared with their experiences in New York: "Allá, en México si uno tiene dinero se ve con doctores, si no, en la casa, con partera" [There, in Mexico, those who have money can be seen by doctors; if not, one's at home with a midwife] (see also Howes-Mischel 2010).

The descriptions of how their mothers and sisters gave birth resembled each other so much, they began to take on the repetitive tones of a mantra, "en la casa," "en el suelo," "con una partera" [at home, on the ground, with a midwife]. Virtually all the women I interviewed described homebirths attended by midwives as the norm for their mother's generation. Those who had given birth to children before migrating described a variety of birth experiences: with midwives, doctors, or nurses; at home, at a midwife's home, at private hospitals, or at public clinics; with anesthesia or other interventions or without; vaginal or caesarean deliveries. Nonetheless, this diversity of experiences was often discursively elided with a dismissive hand gesture, and a statement that one's access to a biomedical birth experience depended on one's economic resources. Most of the women interviewed described themselves as poor prior to migration, and, also, most counted themselves among those excluded from biomedical labor and deliveries. If they did have a baby in a clinic or private hospital, they often went on to point out that this was made possible either by economic advantage ("Gracias a Dios, mi familia tenía los recursos, si no . . ." [Thank God, my family had the means, if not . . .] or by extreme sacrifice ("No teníamos como pagar pero tuvimos que conseguir con mucho sacrificio" [We didn't have a means to pay, but we had to make great sacrifices to get the money]. These "sacrifices" sometimes entailed taking out loans, having money sent from family members in the United States, or establishing payment plans with the clinic or hospital.

Unlike the negative associations that younger women sometimes had with midwife-attended births, the temazcal frequently was described as a loss that women who had migrated felt. In interviews in both New York City and Mexico, discussions of the importance of the temazcal figured prominently. The term is derived from the Nahuatl, *temazcalli*, for heat house; temazcales proliferated throughout pre-Columbian Mesoamerica. Immigrant women from Puebla, Oaxaca, and Guerrero states frequently mentioned temazcales, and it seemed that for some they came to stand for everything that was different about their mother's and grandmothers' birth experiences.

Temazcales are used for steam or dry heat baths and are used prior to conception, during pregnancy, and in the postpartum period, as well as being the location of a host of other therapeutic practices. Many women said that when they had given birth in their home communities, a team comprising their aunts, mother, perhaps sisters and sisters-in-law, partera, or bañera came to collect both mother and child every day for at least a week to bathe them. The mother would be bathed in the temazcal and the baby given a sponge bath in a warm anteroom. Historically, the temazcales were constructed of adobe bricks. More recent temazcal construction is usually of cinderblocks. Many of them can still be seen in small rural towns.[12] Although typically temazcales are for community use, sometimes a household has its own. The center for natural health in Ixtlán de Juárez, Oaxaca, has one in a back room; a low door adjacent to a room for firewood leads to the low-ceilinged brick temazcal still used by parteras. However, in María Pacheco's town, for example, outside of Tehuacán, Puebla, the temazcal fell into disuse years ago. Women told me that, in other towns in rural Mexico with which they were familiar, "el temazcal ya no se usa" [the temazcal is no longer used]. Nonetheless, the liminal period often associated with use of the temazcal remains an important time for caring for the mother and baby.

Lila provided me with a detailed description of temazcal protocols. She had trained as a bañera in her hometown in rural Puebla state. She said that she might have become a partera with more training, but she left to become first a cook at a university in the state capital, then a domestic worker in a diplomatic household in the United States, and thus truncated her practice. I interviewed her at her employer's home (and invitation) in New York City. She said that when a woman has trouble conceiving, she can be treated with a dry heat and smoke bath in a temazcal. While the bath is being prepared, the woman is rubbed with *azufre* (sulfur), alcohol, and a beaten egg. Her waist is tied, and she is given a *polla* to drink, a Coca-Cola stirred with two raw eggs. The *polla* is to help prevent her from fainting from the extreme heat in the bath. She is then wrapped head to toe in sheets and put into the bath for as long as she can stand it, about twenty minutes. If she faints, she might have a bucket of cold water poured on her head to revive her. She sweats out the cold, "suda y saca el frío," and then she is slowly unwrapped over the course of an hour or more as her body acclimates to the outside temperature. One or more *bañeras*, female relatives, and others then bathe her with water and feed her a spoonful of sulfur and an herbal tea. Postpartum mothers are given a similar bath but with a different collection of herbs. They are also given arnica tea to cure their "internal wounds." Following the bath, everyone present may have a beer and perhaps red enchiladas with serrano chiles. A postpartum mother's baby is also feted: blue and white balloons for a boy, pink and white for a girl.

Another of the birth-related practices frequently named in interviews is the use of a *faja*, band, sometimes a *rebozo*, shawl, which is tied around the belly during pregnancy to relieve aches in the back and pelvis, as well as after pregnancy to restore the shape and size of the uterus and abdomen and to expel the air that is said to enter during delivery (see Browner 1985, 486). This wrapping can occur following a session in a temazcal to prevent further exposure to cold air as well as to reshape the uterus. Avoidance of cold, *frío* or *aire*, is one of the key tasks of the attendants in the temazcal as well as all of those who live with the new mother. This is important both in the woman's physical surroundings, to avoid a draft or cooling off too quickly after the vapor bath, and in the food that is ingested, which will be described later (see also Finkler 1994). Violeta, a Oaxaca City–based midwife, told me that aire is dangerous to a nursing mother, who must, when allowing her baby to latch on, ensure that cold air does not get on her nipple or in the baby's open mouth.

Aire is also described as one of the biggest dangers in labor. Prudencia, the midwife in Ixtlán, said that this was one of the factors that led some women to opt for a midwife-attended birth over a biomedical birth in a clinic. Midwives, she said, understood that a woman could not have cold air on her genitals, especially during the liminal period of childbirth. Aire is also reputed to result in protracted labor (Browner 1985, 490). To give birth in a clinic, feet in stirrups with strangers and lights, and genitalia exposed to *los de batas blancas*, the ones in white coats, was viewed as intolerably risky for some women, especially indigenous women, she said. This finding corresponds to Gutmann's report that some traditional midwives described birth in rural Mexican clinics as a rape in which laboring women were stripped of their clothing and family members, shaved, and strapped to sterile metal tables. "Childbirth is thus seen as a biomedical aggression against the mother, and sterile technique as a weapon" (2007, 186). In the births Prudencia attends, women give birth kneeling, with their skirts hanging from around their hips, protecting the baby and their reproductive organs from aire.

Other accounts given to me by women describe the use of a hammock to aid in suspending the laboring woman and giving her a resilient support in a vertical birthing position while the midwife squats in front and other attendants support her from behind. Rebozos might be used to help support a woman or to provide leverage for her to push. Violeta, the midwife in Oaxaca, told me that a woman would be given an herbal preparation so that labor progressed smoothly. A hair might be inserted into her mouth when she was ready to push, "para que le dé asco, y haga fuerza" [so she'll gag and push strongly]. Her belly might be bound with a cloth during labor to support her efforts and squeeze the womb.

Upright positions—kneeling, sitting, squatting, and standing—have been the most common for delivery historically and cross-culturally, favored by practitioners for "privileging the physiology of birth" (Jones 2009, 281). Although in interviews with women living in New York giving birth "en el suelo" [on the floor] came to be one of the most repudiated features of midwife-attended births in Mexico, Prudencia provided a coherent explanation for its purpose—the avoidance of aire. Indeed, women in New York City often remarked to me that they had to "get used to" the idea of a doctor, possibly male, seeing their genitals and of having to open their legs, that it was initially quite discomfiting for them.[13] Floridia, interviewed at the hospital, told me that it was normal in her town to give birth at home "por la pena," because of the embarrassment or shame of displaying one's genitals to strangers. Many of the women interviewed seemed inclined to use different birth postures than the one they were typically permitted in labor and delivery in U.S. hospitals: prostate, with feet in stirrups (Davis-Floyd et al. 2009; van der Geest and Finkler 2004).

After child birth, the *cuarentena* must be respected. The cuarentena was discussed by virtually all my interviewees in each site. Cuarentena is, literally, a quarantine, but in Spanish, as in the word's root language, Latin, it has historically referred to a period of specific duration, forty days, leaving no doubt as to how long isolation is to last (Tyson 2004). It was described in interviews in New York as, at minimum, the requirement that a couple avoid *intimidad,* or *relaciones*, sexual intercourse, for forty days following childbirth. However, most women described a much more elaborate set of practices involving baths, certain foods and beverages, relief from physical labor, and more. During the cuarentena, women were expected to rest, *estar en reposo*, and refrain from all heavy labor and *esfuerzo*, effort, especially sweeping, mopping, and lifting heavy things. To engage in such labor too soon after childbirth could cause hemorrhage and could also contribute to an inadequate healing of the uterus. Because heavy labor can cause wear and tear on a woman's body, it can make future pregnancies difficult; her body might "never" go back to its normal condition.

For a young woman in rural Mexico residing in her mother-in-law's household, the cuarentena may be the only period when she is not expected to do the bulk of household work. On the contrary, it is widely viewed as the mother-in-law's duty to ensure that her daughter-in-law *guarda reposo*, gets her rest, by delegating her work to others. Alma, from Morelos, told me that her suegra took charge of her care during her first pregnancy in Mexico. She contracted a partera for the birth, incurring the wrath of Alma's mother who thought her daughter deserved better. Alma was grateful to her mother-in-law, though, for insisting she keep the cuarentena.

Interestingly, while interviewees in New York described the cuarentena as a decidedly rural, traditional practice that has been slowly chipped away through migration and modernity, Prudencia, the rural Zapotec-speaking midwife, described it as a privilege of the middle class and the urban sphere.[14] She said the largely poor, indigenous women she attends in her hometown wish they could keep the cuarentena but the rigors of their rural life mean that no one can be spared from labor, even temporarily. She said it was her role as a partera to intervene and advocate for new mothers' rights. If a mother-in-law resisted ensuring her daughter-in-law's rest and recovery, the midwife recommended the new mother go to her natal home to be cared for by her own mother. The midwife also scolded husbands who wanted their wives to get back to work right away. She confided to me that, in a city, this would not happen, but in her town, husbands will beat their wives to get them out of bed to make their breakfast.

The practices in rural Mexican towns work not only to heal the new mother but also to provide her a net of social support in the postpartum period. Roberto Castro (2002) writes about the hierarchical social relations in the town of Ocuituco, Morelos, in which younger women are at the bottom of the social universe. Patriarchal relations, patrilineal descent, and virilocality are forces promoting the circulation and possession of women as the property of their husband's households, and thus they enjoy fewer opportunities than young men to study, work outside the home, move about freely, control their fertility and sexuality, and more.[15] Practices like the cuarentena have historically mitigated the sexual, labor, and other demands placed on young women. It enables them a short-lived but culturally sanctioned respite from their obligations and a certain degree of pampering. Within these practices, specialists like the partera enjoy legitimacy in intervening in domestic relations to protect their clients and to help them to recover from childbirth.

In the postpartum period, women said they are advised to avoid certain foods and to consume others. Violeta recommends *caldo de gallo de días*, soup made with a days-old rooster, for healing and promoting milk production. Many women mentioned *atole*, a thick, cornstarch-based drink, as highly recommended for postpartum mothers. Women interviewed described familiarity with an elaborate system of desirable "hot" foods and prohibited "cold" foods. This regime corresponds to complex notions about humoral-balance restoration in Mesoamerican pregnancy and childbirth practices (Cosminsky 1982; Finkler 1994; Jordan 1993; Masley 2007, 26). Pork usually topped the list of prohibited foods. Virtually all women said warm tortillas, hot chocolate, and toasted bread were good for women following labor. In addition, Violeta recommended beer or *pulque*, a fermented corn drink, to stimulate milk production (Masley 2007, 29).

In Oaxaca, Violeta said that when a boy is born, the family may invite all the attendants and neighbors to feast on a goat, *chivo*. For a girl, the party is more modest, perhaps a bean stew, because a girl is considered to have less economic potential. Midwives are also paid differently, as much as one thousand Mexican pesos for a boy, two hundred for a girl, I was told by one Oaxacan midwife.[16] In today's context of migration, *padrinos*, godparents or festive cosponsors, are called on to chip in for celebrations like baptisms and weddings. In the Bronx, Josefina invited me to her house to watch her wedding video, a several hours-long tape that included both the ceremony and the party, with long takes focused on the serving of the goat meat by female relatives and neighbors. I asked who had been invited to the wedding feast: "todos, pues, todo el pueblo" [everyone, of course, the whole town]. Such a grand party in today's dollarized economy is typically possible only through contributions by members of the family working in the United States (see also Pauli 2008).

While postpartum women are treated to herbal baths, teas, and unctures, their babies are likewise lavished with attention from their elder female kin.

The importance of this care-giving practice was especially poignant for María Pacheco, who, as we will see in the next chapter, contrasts what she thinks would have happened had she given birth in her hometown with the reality: when she was alone, recovering from labor in a Bronx apartment and experiencing postpartum depression, she wanted nothing more than for someone she could trust to take the baby off her hands for an hour. Many women who felt they had properly respected the cuarentena reported rapid and thorough recovery from childbirth, and some boasted that their body showed no signs of having had a child.

The Changing Landscape of Care

Although the practices described thus far in this chapter are the ones most frequently cited by the New York–based research participants, these women migrated, on average, 6.5 years before our interviews, in the late 1990s–2000. Consequently, the pregnancy and childbirth practices they remember may no longer be prevalent today. In this section, interviews in Oaxaca with a mother and daughter who are a lay midwife and medical doctor, respectively, illustrate some of the ways that the landscape of birth practices is changing in Mexico at the same time that the lives of Mexican immigrant women have also changed.

I sat talking with Teresa (called Tere) and her mother, Violeta, in Violeta's sunny, flower-filled home abutting a creek in the neighborhood of Oaxaca called Río Blanco.[17] Tere sat on a sofa with me, playing with her year-old daughter at the same time, but Violeta seemed incapable of taking a seat. She roasted tomatoes for a salsa on the stove-top, folded laundry, began a new load of laundry in the washer outside, started to stew something in a pot, spoke with a son who stepped in briefly, poured water on some potted flowers, and periodically chimed in with her opinions and comments. I was eager to speak with both women: Tere is a young doctor in general practice in Oaxaca City, and Violeta is a partera with decades of experience. Both seemed to assume that Tere's and my proximity in age and life stage (as mothers of young children) as well as high levels of education would mean that her historical, medical, and social explanations would be of more use to me, an anthropologist. This sort of dynamic mirrored the way that the two described their perspectives on prenatal care and childbirth. Both women gave Tere's expertise obtained through medical school greater authority. Even while Violeta's "empirical" knowledge was honored and esteemed by both, it was discursively made to recede into the background, secondary to scientific approaches. This dynamic between mother and daughter bears many similarities to a larger process by which longstanding care practices associated with pregnancy and childbirth have come to be marginalized and, in some cases, displaced entirely by biomedical, scientific approaches. This changing epistemology surrounding reproduction has a significant impact on the ways women experience pregnancy and childbirth in Mexico and among Mexicans in the United States.

Tere completed her year of practical training as a doctor in San Juan Bautista Tuxtepec, a rural town north of the state capital of Oaxaca. In addition to her work as a midwife, Violeta also had the personal experience of having given birth to eleven children of her own, without complications. The two marveled at each other's knowledge, and each saw the other's expertise as complementary to her own. Tere said her mother was an expert whose wisdom and practical experience could never be achieved from book study. At the same time, Violeta was proud of her daughter's academic accomplishments and professional status. Tere said that while she was in medical school her mother would invite her along to visit her pregnant clients so that she could provide a "technical explanation" for what was happening to their bodies. In turn, when Tere was completing her internship, Violeta went to Tuxtepec to visit her and saw "una chica que tuvo su bebé con partera en una situación insalubre" [a girl who'd had her baby with a midwife in an unsanitary situation]. The husband had insisted that his wife have their baby with the same midwife who had delivered his mother's babies. Tere recounted, "Mi mamá vio los riesgos, que el niño tuvo fiebre, por falta de higiene" [My mother saw the risks, that the child had a fever because of a lack of hygiene]. Tere went on to describe midwives who work clandestinely because they do not wish to become certified, who do not speak Spanish, or who inject their clients in the buttocks with oxytocin to induce labor: "Eso no se puede hacer, eso se tiene que introducir de manera entrevenosa, ocho gotas por hora" [That cannot be; that medicine has to be administered on an intravenous drip, eight drops per hour].

Even while she hailed her mother's rapport with her clients and expertise in herbal preparations for inducing labor, preventing hemorrhage, increasing milk production, "composing" the uterus, and more, she turned her description of her own training as a doctor into an object lesson about the ways that advances in biomedical technology save lives. She rhetorically elicited her mother's agreement with the superiority of a hygienic, scientific, technical approach to childbirth that could be enriched and enhanced by traditional knowledge and practices. Tere also remarked that she was one of the few members of her cohort who understood the contributions parteras empíricas have made and the knowledge they hold.[18] She yearned for more of the parteras to become certified so they could be partners in the project of delivering healthy babies and lowering infant and maternal mortality.

When it came time for Tere to deliver her own baby, she went to the hospital where she had completed her medical training. She said she had her baby "normally," in that she did not have a cesarean, but that she needed to be induced because she did not go into labor on her own and "porque era estrecha de cadera" [because she had narrow hips], a common explanation given for interventions during labor by women I interviewed in New York. She was not charged for the birth, although she said that prior to a recently implemented government program, Arranque Parejo de la Vida [Fair Start in Life], which eliminated charges for birth, labor and delivery in a hospital typically cost four thousand pesos (see Secretaría de la Salud 2002).

When I asked her whether she kept the cuarentena, she associated it with complete bed rest and told me that in fact it was not recommended: "Si una mujer está acostada, perjudica la circulación, la sangre se estanca y se pueden dar trombos" [If a woman is lying down, she limits her circulation, the blood pools up and she can get clots]. She said she negotiates the concept of the need for a forty-day period of rest as a doctor by telling patients that forty days is about the time it takes for a woman to stop bleeding after childbirth, a sign she can go back to all of her usual routines: "Así es como médicamente manejamos la cuarentena" [That is how we medically manage *la cuarentena*].

"Indigenous medicine" in Mexico has long had to negotiate with the certifying and authorizing apparatuses of the state and with the forces of colonization, and, later, with globalization (Alatorre Wynter 1990; Finkler 2004). In pre-Columbian central Mexico and many other regions of Mesoamerica the healing arts were closely linked with ritual specialists (Pérez Loredo Díaz 1991). Parteras' expertise was sought out not only for pregnancy care and labor and delivery but even for matchmaking advice prior to a couple's union. They used both mundane and mystical strategies in caring for their clients. Spanish colonists often marveled at the extensive knowledge and skills of healing specialists, called *ticitl* in Nahuatl, including parteras, or *temixhihuatiani* (Alatorre Wynter 1990, 75). Colonial doctors also adopted many of the practices of indigenous healing specialists (Finkler 2004, 2040). Bernardino de Sahagún wrote extensively about the work of these specialists in the Florentine Codex ([1561–1582] 1950). However, the more spiritual aspects of their work were quickly demonized as witchcraft and subject to the punitive attentions of the Inquisition (Alatorre Wynter 1990, 76).

Meanwhile, obstetrics was, in the colonial period, considered a base specialization among Spanish doctors. While ritual specialists were driven out and replaced by Catholic priests, and other ticitl by surgeons and other practitioners, the Spanish colonists did not count in their numbers many people who knew how to deliver babies or, much less, cared to. Attention to pregnant and laboring women, both indigenous and Spanish, continued to be a largely home-based practice left to indigenous parteras after independence and until the end of the nineteenth century. Further, parteras retained and in fact probably enhanced their highly regarded status in their communities throughout and following the colonial period—a status that, in some cases, they would retain until the present.

Alatorre Wynter notes that it was only in 1972, when the federal government ordered that any institution offering courses in surgery and general medicine also had to offer training to lay midwives, that midwifery would be genuinely threatened in Mexico. Ironically, Alatorre Wynter notes, midwifery gained status and prestige as it became a topic of legitimate study in the academy, and thus "en el cirujano se encontraba el embrión del futuro partero en México y que, al asumir la responsabilidad de ejercer la obstericia, inicia una lucha contra la partera hasta lograr muchos años después, su extinction" [in the surgeon is found the embryo of the future midwife (masculine noun) in Mexico, who, on assuming the responsibility of practicing obstetrics, began a struggle that would finally, many years later, result in the midwife's (feminine noun) extinction] (1990, 77; see also Finkler 2004).

Prudencia, the rural Oaxaca midwife, described the economy of state-certified midwifery. Although she obtained legal certification to practice as a lay midwife, Prudencia incurred a great deal of debt to do so. Further, although her hometown, which she described as far more rural and remote than Ixtlán de Juárez, itself a small, remote town with respect to the state capital, did not have a public clinic, her midwifery business was not booming in its absence. To make ends meet, she sought shifts of several days' duration at the natural health center in Ixtlán. Although babies were not delivered there, she used the temazcal for steam baths, administered sobadas, gave consultations, and promoted her own and others' herbal lotions and unguents.

Although parteras have yet to become extinct and by some measures are experiencing a renaissance, their work has been considerably circumscribed. Midwives deliver fewer babies, but they have received new and expanded roles in efforts of the federal health service to incorporate (some say co-opt) traditional medicine within Western biomedical spaces and practices. Further, midwives and other healing specialists have joined the burgeoning industry of traditional medicine marketed to the large expatriate and tourist population in Oaxaca City and other places in Mexico; services include thermal baths, sobadas, *limpias* (spiritual cleansings), and any number of other healing practices. Today, in Oaxaca City, one most frequently sees temazcales in the guise of temazcal-spas, New Age–style therapeutic saunas frequented by foreigners as well as some elite Mexicans, part of what Gutmann calls "indigenous medical tourism" (2007, 193; also Maldonado 2010b).

The Mexican national health service has expanded its reach into virtually all rural communities. Medical students, finished with coursework and ready to begin practice, like Tere, staff these spare rural clinics, sometimes single-handedly, and this intense immersion into public health is viewed as the final step in their training as well as a service obligation. This expansion of public clinics is part of a massive federal effort to reduce maternal and infant mortality. Tere informed me that in addition to staffing the clinics and serving their host community's immediate medical needs, the young doctors are required to con-duct a census of women of childbearing age as well as of midwives. The purpose of the census is to prescribe folic acid to all women older than twelve years of age as a prophylactic for birth defects, to distribute information regarding *plani-ficación familiar,* family planning, and sexually transmitted diseases, and to urge all pregnant women to begin or to continue prenatal care. Women who have reached *paridez satisfecha,* desired parity, are encouraged to have a tubal ligation. The doctors also identify midwives as part of a related effort to certify them.

These efforts are only the most recent in a larger process of medicalization of pregnancy and childbirth in Mexico. Claudia, born in 1983 in Castillotla, Puebla, said she and her siblings were born in a clinic. She said that there the attendants "son más preparados, tienen más experiencia, está más desarrol-lado. Ya no se usan las parteras" [are more prepared, they have more experience; it is more developed. Now midwives are no longer used]. Use of traditional care practices is viewed by many women in this study as a function of necessity, not desire or as one option among others available to them, much less to their mothers and grandmothers.

However, although the landscape of care practices is changing, it is not changing uniformly in the direction of increased medicalization.[19] For Mexico to fully equip every small municipality with a clinic and certified personnel, including trained birth attendants, not only is prohibitively expensive but is more in keeping with the social safety net promoted by more progressive politi-cal parties than the Partido de Acción Nacional (PAN), which took control of the presidency in 2000 and between 1997 and 2010 gained a significant num-ber of congressional seats, state governorships, and local offices. Instead, a neoliberal emphasis on privatization as well as on self-care and "vigilance" has accompanied continued efforts to provide minimal state-funded health care and nonmedical care approaches under a framework of "choice" (Maldonado 2010b; Smith-Oka 2009). We can trace midwifery and traditional medicine within this political timeline. After decades of marginalizing traditional birth practices as part of efforts to "modernize" health care, in the early 1980s Mexico began to move toward accommodation of some components of traditional medicine, especially herbalism and midwifery (Sesia 1996, 122). Perhaps the most overt act of this accommodation was a decree by the state of Oaxaca in 2001 that traditional medicine was to be recognized as an equal of biomedical, or allopathic, medicine (Gutmann 2007, 167). Eduardo Menéndez attributes such openness to the "primarily empirical and technical nature of these practices which health authorities believe is easily reducible to the scientific rationale that supports the biomedical model without threatening the ideology or hegemony of the biomedical care system" (quoted in Sesia 1996, 122).[20]

Since 1990, midwives who are found operating without certification are told that they must enroll in a certification course or cease to practice. The certification courses are time-consuming and may involve fees and expenses, including travel to an urban center. To transfer knowledge that has been gained through embodied practice into exams is antithetical, if not virtually impossible for some midwives, who frequently have had little formal schooling and who have sometimes been delivering babies for longer than young doctors have been alive. They frequently find being asked to do so annoying if not offensive (Alatorre Wynter 1994; Sesia 1996).[21]

Although some doctors and some media reports cheerfully praise the ambitious reach of the federal government's public health campaign and its efforts to bring the Mexican countryside "into the twenty-first century," for many midwives the campaign has sounded the death knell for their practice. Told they could have legal problems if they continue to deliver babies without certification, many midwives have opted to cease practicing. In addition to the unfortunate demise of a vast amount of knowledge, their withdrawal from practicing has generated some social problems. Midwives are reputed to be unable to deny a request for assistance by a pregnant woman or her family, and even payment for such services is sometimes thought to violate their ethical obligation to attend anyone who needs them. Thus, Violeta told me, midwives who have decided to cease practicing are put in the uncomfortable position of either refusing to deliver a baby against their assumed longstanding moral obligation to do so or they deliver babies clandestinely, risking legal trouble and also difficulties if a laboring woman requires an emergency transfer to a medical facility. Future research could be fruitfully conducted to explore how the decision of some midwives to cease practicing may have produced conflicts and ethical dilemmas in their communities.

Some midwives view their decision to cease practicing as an acceptance of the inevitable changing of the times. When I interviewed her, Violeta continued to provide herbal remedies, massage, and consultations, but she stated that she only occasionally delivered babies and that when she did, it was often as a last resort when a family "failed" to obtain proper prenatal care. Tere gave the example of a young woman in her neighborhood who had eclampsia, which she defined for me as convulsions that can follow from untreated preeclampsia, pregnancy-induced hypertension. She said the young woman had not sought prenatal care and that when she went into labor, she was rushed to a clinic where her baby was delivered at 1.5 kilos (3.3 pounds). The young woman was left disabled, unable to speak, walk, or use the bathroom alone. Tere described the young woman's case as a result of ignorance and poverty: the young woman and her mother are vendors at a local street market, *tianguis*, and according to Tere's account, the mother felt she could not spare her daughter for prenatal care visits.

Some specialists complain that their practice was co-opted by the new federal regulations and they were reduced to being messengers of a fertility-control campaign by the government, expected to promote contraceptives among their clientele (Organización de Médicos Indígenas de la Mixteca 2009). Further, Violeta and Prudencia explained that, given the choice, many of their former patients or the daughters of their former patients opted for a clinic or hospital birth and no longer sought out a midwife.

Even though many midwives no longer deliver babies, they say that parteras and brujos remain key figures for many pregnant women. They say that even when present a doctor *que está de pasante*, only in town temporarily, will not usually enjoy the same close relationships with community members that characterize a partera's role (see Gutmann 2007, 167–169). Violeta and Tere said that even in towns with a medical clinic the lay midwives sometimes retain greater authority and trust than the doctors at the clinic because of their long-standing relationships in the community. Further, although more births occur in clinics today, many women prefer to address other aspects of pregnancy and postpartum care with parteras and other specialists. In an earlier study, Browner reported that in spite of the installation of public health centers, rural-community dwellers in the town where she conducted her research continued to prefer herbal remedies for reproduction-related health problems (1985, 484).

Neoliberal Health Care Reforms and Locating Responsibility for Care

In contemporary discourses about the responsibilities of the state to its citizens, access to biomedical care during pregnancy and childbirth is often cast as a human right. This is the language used to describe the programs under which the federal government of Mexico is funding the extension of free prenatal care and delivery to rural areas. Many women denigrate the birth experiences of their mothers and grandmothers in Mexico as characteristic of poverty and a corrupt and weak federal government.

Mexico's government frames prenatal care and childbirth largely as a measure of the country's modernity and aspirations to join the top tier of industrialized nations. Progress toward the goal of having a healthy, modern nation-state is indicated in part by the maternal mortality rate, which has been called "a public health problem not only in comparison with other developed and developing countries." Public health professionals insist that "a significant number of deaths could be avoided with high-quality care during pregnancy and childbirth" (Langer and Hernández 2002, 4), a view shared by the Mexican government, which has identified the reduction of maternal mortality as one of its principal goals (President of the Republic of Mexico 2009), in keeping with Millennium Development Goal 6, to improve maternal health (United Nations 2000). Mexico's maternal mortality rate has dropped dramatically, from 100 of every 100,000 live births between 1945 and 1960, to 39 in 2000 (Velasco 2002).[22] Although the United Nations describes the reduction of maternal mortality as requiring a multifaceted effort centered on increasing the number of skilled birth attendants, increasing access to emergency obstetric care, increasing access to contraception (which it says could reduce maternal mortality by 30 percent), and reducing adolescent pregnancy, Mexico's approach is more narrow, stressing "universal attention for pregnancy complications and [promotion of] a culture of risk prevention and self-care among pregnant women" (President of the Republic of Mexico 2009).

In a report commissioned and distributed by the Instituto Mexicano del Seguro Social (IMSS), researchers described efforts to lower Mexico's maternal mortality as centering on three basic conditions: providing universal and accessible medical care, educating women to use these services, and improving the quality of prenatal and hospital-based obstetric care (Velasco 2002, 2). It is relevant to note that the term used for prenatal care in the report is *vigilance*: "calidad adecuada de la vigilancia prenatal" [adequate quality of prenatal vigilance]; this phrasing implies that pregnancy is a dangerous and complication-prone pathology requiring medical supervision. The report puts a strong emphasis on education and the responsibility of mothers for the health of their pregnancies. This emphasis is ironic, given that until the turn of the century, poor rural women largely had little choice but to care for themselves with lay midwives because of the lack of other care options. In another article in the same report, two doctors write that maternal mortality can be reduced through concrete interventions into specific areas that they call "los tres retrasos" [the three delays]: delays in obtaining medical attention and recognizing an obstetric complication, delays in getting to a site where care can be obtained, and delays in obtaining timely care on arrival at such a site (Langer and Hernández 2002, 4).

Terms like *vigilance* further evoke the relationship between modern nation-states and surveillance, as in Michel Foucault's notion of "governmentality," in which knowledge about and technologies of surveillance pragmatically guide and regulate everyday life (1991). In this way, the obligation of graduating medical students to conduct censuses in rural communities of pregnant women, midwives, and women of childbearing age in order to prescribe them folic acid, offer family planning advice, and ensure that midwives are certified falls squarely within Foucauldian understandings of the bureaucratic modern state, in which knowledge is power. In the ideal modern state, knowledge contributes to self-regulation so that violence need not be overt and citizens manage and enforce their own compliance with norms. Vigilance is thus inextricably linked to "self-care." Aihwa Ong describes this connection as neoliberal governmentality: "the concepts that inform the government of free individuals who are then induced to self-manage according to market principles of discipline, efficiency and competitiveness" (2006, 4). Maldonado writes about the increasing emphasis on self-care by the state in contemporary Mexico as a feature of neoliberal policy in which citizens are consumers largely responsible for caring for themselves in the absence of comprehensive state-subsidized care (2010b).

Under the constraints of international monetary policy in the mid-1990s, the ruling party, the Partido Revolucionario Institucional (PRI), withdrew state services in a marked fashion. With the decidedly more neoliberal approach of the PAN, the presidencies of Vicente Fox and Felipe Calderón continued even further down that path. As Napolitano writes, "Modernization without real democracy has its toll. Throughout [Carlos] Salinas Gotari's presidency and partly during President [Ernesto] Zedillo's term, a de facto withdrawal of the state's food, health and educational programs (also imposed on the Mexican government by International Monetary Fund rescue plans) has weakened the safety net that existed for a good part of the Mexican low-income population" (2002, 14). The safety net is even weaker today than it was then in much of the republic.

The overall framing of maternal mortality is thus one of vigilance, self-care, and overcoming delays. Responsibility for healthy pregnancies is handed back to mothers. *Retraso* is translated as delay, but it has a secondary meaning of backwardness. There is no separating Mexico's public health care policies from its overall project to achieve the status of a first-tier industrialized nation. This teleological stance toward modernity necessarily implies an "overcoming" of the retrasos that are hindering progress. This goal is echoed in broader state projects as well. Oaxaca's state slogan, for example, is "Oaxaca, de cara a la nación" [facing the nation], and its website reads, "Hablar de transformación es hablar de Oaxaca" [To speak of transformation is to speak of Oaxaca] (Gobierno del Estado de Oaxaca 2009). This slogan bears interesting correlations to the discourse of superación, a word that also implies overcoming, and provides a partial explanation for common perceptions of the medicalization of pregnancy and childbirth care as a sign of modernity. Vania Smith-Oka describes these federal efforts as deriving from a sort of national inferiority complex: "The Mexican government has had deep-seated fears of underdevelopment and over-population of the poor. It has identified contraception as the ideal means to modernize Mexico and move away from 'stereotypical' behaviors, including having too many children" (2009, 2070).

Within this kind of framing, parteras must be assimilated into the larger federal health system. Their role is one of supplementing and lending credibil-ity to the medical providers whose approach is cast as superior, more techno-logical and science-based than "traditional" approaches, which are seen as a necessary, if inadequate, recourse in the absence of a robust public health sys-tem. In this way, Violeta, convinced of the need for a "hygienic" environment for birth with a professionally trained attendant, such as her daughter, happily makes way for a new, more advanced system; her empirical knowledge is help-ful but largely obsolete and irrelevant to the outcome of birth.

On May 28, 2009, International Women's Health Day, Mexican President Calderón announced a new federal policy making any woman eligible to receive care free of charge at any clinic or hospital of the Instituto de Seguridad y Servicios Sociales de los Trabajadores del Estado (ISSTE), the IMSS, or the Health Secretariat, regardless of her membership in any of these organizations (President of the Republic of Mexico 2009). This policy followed on the expan-sion of public health care provision through IMSS-Oportunidades.[23] IMSS-Oportunidades extends basic medical care throughout the republic through the work of 16,620 doctors, nurses, and paramedics as well as 287,000 volunteer health promoters in a network called Modelo de Atención Integral a la Salud, Integrated Model of Health Care. This is the system in which Tere completed her practical training. These initiatives have their work cut out for them. Puebla, Oaxaca, and Guerrero, of Mexico's thirty-one states, are among the six with the lowest rates of births in a public or private institution, some of the highest rates of maternal mortality, and the lowest rates of coverage by the major health care providers: IMSS and ISSTE (Secretaría de la Salud 2002; see also Howes-Mischel 2010).

The location of responsibility for care of pregnant women and the institutional framework and specialists in and by which care is disbursed are shifting rapidly in rural and urban Mexico. The efforts of the federal government to address high rates of maternal and infant mortality have led to a reorganization of care provision, at the same time that neoliberal structural adjustment has implied an ever-limited public budget for such care. The supplantation of "empirical midwives" and other traditional medical specialists by doctors in training and certification regimes has made clear that, for the federal government, biomedical, technoscientific models of care, even when administered by inexpert providers, is superior to previous, home-based models of traditional care. Although data-based recommendations such as the U.N. Millennium Development Goals make clear that birth is safest with a "skilled birth attendant," the assumption that such skills count only when possessed by a medical doctor in training or a midwife who has completed certification courses is an indicator more of the technoscientific bias of the state's apparatus of certification than of the efficacy of traditional, empirical midwifery.

Moreover, the state is not an entity exclusive of the people that constitute the nation, and the valorization of biomedical approaches is not an exclusive domain of the federal government's policymakers. On the contrary, there is a powerful popular demand for biomedical care and a concomitant view by many that traditional care practices have historically constituted a less than preferred adaptation to poverty. Further, neoliberal articulations of citizenship, arguably a product of the shrinkage of progressive models of governance, offer their own allure to individuals. Migrating to the United States to access higher-paying labor opportunities and hospital-based health care is an expression of neoliberal ideals of self: flexible, self-sufficient, and mobile. In the congruence of what the state and its ever diminishing resource base requires of citizens and what citizens themselves want we may find the reasons many Mexican immigrant women are enthusiastic about the care they receive in New York hospitals, even while that care implies a rupture of what many of them thought they knew about pregnancy. Further, the shifting locations in which families make their lives mean that changes that have occurred to the care landscape in their home communities may go unremarked because so many people have opted to remove themselves through migration.

Chapter 4

Becoming Patients

Birth Experiences in New York City

If María Pacheco had given birth to her daughter in her childhood home in a small rural municipality outside of Tehuacán, Puebla, her mother told me she would have been treated to forty days of *reposo*, rest, during the cuarentena. During that time of recuperation, her mother, sister, sisters-in-law, and mother-in-law would have bathed her in hot herbal steam baths, bound her womb with a rebozo, cooked appropriate "hot" foods for her, and given her special herbal teas to *componer*, literally compose or repair, her insides as well as increase her milk production. Although her small town no longer has a temazcal or a practicing midwife, her return from the local government clinic would have been marked by a whole range of practices designed to care for and aid the recovery and bonding of mother and baby. Sitting in her cheerful kitchen lit by the intense Puebla sun, her mother told me the names of the herbs she had at the ready for such treatments and expressed sorrow that her daughter had been far away when she had her babies.

Instead, María spent the day after giving birth alone in a hospital room, her baby shuttled off to the nursery and her husband gone to work. She cried all day long, the beginning of a severe bout of postpartum depression. After she and the baby came home, her husband, Raúl, would rise before dawn to cook chicken soup and rice for her and leave it ready on the stove before going off to his job as a busboy. She stayed in their bedroom, out of sight of Raúl's male cousins, their housemates, sobbing and resisting the urge to spank or ignore her screaming newborn. When Raúl told María's mother over the phone that she was covered in a rash, depressed, bleeding profusely, and still unable to nurse, her mother sent herbs with a cousin who was traveling to New York City and

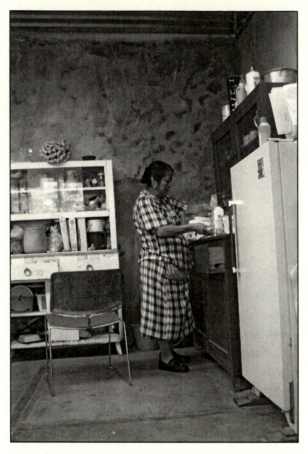

Figure 4   María Pacheco's mother in her kitchen, August 2008. Photo by the author.

instructed Raúl how to boil the herbs and imitate a steam bath in their apartment bathtub by using boiling water from a tea kettle. He obtained some cin-
derblock bricks that he stacked in the tub, and she sat on them, cloaked in a
sheet, cautious not to touch the boiling water he poured around the bricks and
over the herbs.

The separation between María and the kinship network that would have
helped her in this difficult period was produced by María and Raul's migration
but also was exacerbated by the undocumented nature of it. Even if the couple
had the money to send for María's mother, she was unlikely to get a visa, and,
as an undocumented immigrant, María could not visit Mexico. Immigration
laws and their immigrant circumstances made the birth of a child, by custom
an event rejoiced over and attended to by an extensive network of kin, into a

lonely task that the couple fumbled through alone. By taking on the role of his mother, mother-in-law, and sister-in-law, not only did Raúl get María through a tough period, but also their bond was strengthened (see Hirsch 2003). Their struggles confirm their idea of themselves as a couple: a lonely unit of mutual support and affection, facing the struggles and challenges of life as migrants. This image corresponds to contemporary conceptualizations of companionate marriage, premised on romance, affection, respect, and partnership between two spouses, "characterized by sexual and emotional intimacy and somewhat less hierarchical relations between the sexes" (Hirsch et al. 2010, 10; Hirsch 2003). Although the couple's relationship was strengthened by Raúl's willingness to do what only female kin would have done in their hometown, María does not look back fondly on the first weeks she spent with her daughter. On the contrary, one of her biggest fears when she was pregnant with her second child, nearly seven years later, was that she would have to go through the same kind of experience again.

In this chapter, I explore the birth and pregnancy experiences of Mexican immigrant women in New York City as they move through the public health care system and after they come home. In the first research phase of this study, at the community center in Queens where I conducted interviews and participant observation, women told me about their experiences in hospitals throughout the city. One woman, Nancy, told me that she walked in early labor to Elmhurst Hospital from her home in Jackson Heights, more than two miles away, with her husband and toddler. She was told that there was nowhere for her child to wait for her in the hospital (in contrast to birthing centers and hospitals that have family waiting rooms). Because the couple did not have others they trusted to care for their toddler during her labor, the husband went home with their son, amid promises from the nurses that they would phone him when his wife was ready to deliver. Not only did they not call her husband, but Nancy went through what she described as an excruciating labor alone, with only intermittent checks of her status by nurses. No one accompanied or coached her during labor. When she felt an urge to push and desperately called out for assistance, a nurse told her she could not, that the doctor was not ready. Although she tried not to, to refrain from pushing when a fetus is "crowning" is virtually impossible. She told me the nurses scolded her, telling her that she could not have her baby until the doctor arrived. Ultimately, she delivered her baby utterly alone, abandoned even by the nurse who had gone to look for the obstetrician in attendance.

Other women told me of verbal insults and humiliations and a rampant lack of translation services in other hospitals around the city. Even so, Gabriela told me that for her it was precisely a lack of Spanish-speaking personnel that made Manhattan Hospital a good site for receiving health care. She opted for Manhattan in part because she had heard that Manhattan had fewer Spanish-speaking personnel than there were at Elmhurst Hospital in Queens, where she had delivered her first child. She said, "La atención acá [Manhattan Hospital] es diferente. Allá, hay muchos hispanos que trabajan y entre los mismos hispanos nos tratamos mal. Aquí hay menos hispanos. Nos brinda más confianza. No se enojan tanto" [Here, the attention one is given is different. There, there are many Hispanic workers, and among Hispanics we treat each other poorly. Here there are fewer Hispanics. This gives us more confidence. They don't get as angry.] When I asked two sisters, Marta and Isabel, about their experiences with childbirth, they raved about the wonderful labor and delivery experiences they had at Manhattan with midwives. I was impressed, as they were the only women I had interviewed to that date who had delivered with midwives in New York City. And, thus, Marta and Isabel prompted my pursuit of Manhattan Hospital's prenatal clinic as a research site.

Subjectification and Superación: The Prenatal Clinic

"Mexican patients really organize as families to care for a pregnant mother. The lady who cleans for me, when she became pregnant, stopped working and stayed home taking care of her sister's kids and her sister cleaned for me. Then when the sister got pregnant, they switched." This quotation is from a certified nurse-midwife (CNM) who attends patients in the public prenatal clinic where I conducted research. She clearly holds positive views toward the Mexican patients in her care. Nonetheless, her comment is remarkably anecdotal for a provider of prenatal care to many Mexican immigrant patients. This midwife sees as many as twenty-five patients in a day, about a quarter of them Mexican. She and her midwifery colleagues were observed by me to be among the most caring, warm, and generous prenatal providers I encountered in the course of research and received praise from their patients in interviews. Why then would she cite a domestic employee as a source of data when in her professional experience she has hundreds of patients to whom she might have referred? This is an example of the impersonal dynamic of the public prenatal clinic, in which, in spite of almost constant interaction, providers and patients may never get to know one another and instead make frequent and even dangerous assumptions about each other.

For the most part, Mexican immigrant women described being treated well in large, oversubscribed, and underfunded Manhattan Hospital. In fact, many women said in interviews that they chose this hospital after using other hospitals in which they felt they had been mistreated. Medical settings are one of the sites most named by migrants as places where they have experienced discrimination (Massey and Sánchez 2010, 130), but most women in this study did not recount experiencing it at Manhattan Hospital. The fact that the vast majority of the women served in the clinic do not live in Manhattan and travel long distances to receive prenatal care there is one testament to its good reputation. For their part, Mexican patients are often treated in this hospital as "model patients" for their diligence with keeping appointments, their docility, and their low rates of high-risk behaviors (such as alcohol and substance abuse). One midwife told me, "We love Mexican patients. That's why we love working here. They're so healthy." Other groups are sometimes unfavorably compared to Mexican patients.[1] Nonetheless, several features of the prenatal care administered even in this rather well-functioning clinical setting contributed to processes of "subjectification" of prenatal patients (Ong 1996), a disciplining of them into certain types of behavior and attitudes that did not spare Mexican patients. At the same time, Mexican immigrant patients frequently enter the prenatal care arena as part of their own project of superación, which began with their migration. The intersection of two very different processes, subjectification and superación, can be toxic in ways that the women, and certainly the providers too, may not realize until it is too late.

The prenatal clinic is, in many ways, a model of organizational management. Although it is oversubscribed and underfunded, typically, pregnant patients do not have to wait long to get a prenatal appointment or to be seen when they arrive. The clinic is organized to see a maximum number of patients with a minimum of resources. At this clinic, low-risk pregnancies are routinely attended by CNMs, and only high-risk pregnancies are uniformly supervised by obstetricians. Thus, the midwives see the vast majority of patients, and on any given morning a stack of thirty to forty pink charts await them. The team of three to four midwives has about three hours to work its way through the stack before lunch; a new stack of thirty to forty charts then appears. Medical assistants organize the charts and call patients in, weigh them, process their urine samples, take vitals, and then send them into a holding room where midwives collect them for a seven- to ten-minute private examination. Medical assistants also run the reception desk, so, depending on their shift, they handle one or another section of a vast assembly line of care. All patients are referred to as "mami," and they are funneled through the clinic's rooms efficiently with generic warmth. There is little space within this system for meaningful interaction. Providers and patients may never see each other again as assignment of patients is random each visit. The seven minutes allotted to exams allows little time for patients and providers to talk off script. After the initial visit, in which women detail their reproductive histories, almost no time is spent on the prior experiences or knowledge women bring to their pregnancies. Frequently, my interviews with patients revealed vast amounts of information about their pregnancy histories and practices for caring for themselves during pregnancy that had no place in the prenatal encounter; there was no opportunity for such information to be revealed, let alone recorded. Although midwives gathered interesting "anecdotes" chatting with patients, frequently while escorting them out of the room, and sometimes recounted these to me later, these stories seemed never to emerge in patients' charts or to affect their care.

As they are moved through the system over the course of their pregnancies, patients' attitudes, knowledge, and experience rarely come to be known by their providers. Instead, their "risk profile" plays a large role in the tone and quality of treatment they receive. Although identification of the risk factors associated with pathological health outcomes is one of the great achievements of contemporary epidemiology, when deployed in clinical encounters, it can have a deleterious effect on the way patients are treated and, ultimately, on their health outcomes. Risk profiles are an epistemological technology of control: the care and treatment protocols of patients are built largely on their risk profiles, as sometimes also are the attitudes of providers toward them. Obstetrician Bethany Hays writes, "In medicine, in order to maintain the illusion of control, we learn to treat the *potential* for problems as a problem" (1996, 293). Although this might be good medical practice if risk factors were more exactly correlated with pathology, such calculations can be only as precise as the most current research, which is constantly being shown to have tremendous blind spots and faults (Palloni and Morenoff 2001).

At the same time that they receive prenatal "care," Mexican immigrant patients receive particular messages about appropriate behaviors and expected attitudes and are treated by providers in accordance with their perceived compliance with new regimes of comportment. In public prenatal care settings immigrant women's own narratives and desires to superarse clash with discourses about immigrants as a drain on public resources, ill-equipped for self-care, and noncompliant, even while some providers speak of Mexican women as "model patients." When poor immigrant women access care in a public prenatal clinic, they are initiated into a series of intrusive processes by which they establish and retain eligibility for services (see Bridges, 2011, 93). Nikolas Rose and Carlos Novas write that "new biological and biomedical languages are beginning to 'make up citizens' in new ways in the deliberations, calculations, and strategies of experts and authorities" (2005, 445). In this way, any interaction with the state, whether in a bureaucratic realm or, arguably, even more so in the medico-bureaucratic sphere of a public hospital, has as its result the production of new subjectivities, new formulations of citizenship.

New York State subsidizes prenatal care for poor women, irrespective of migratory status. Thus, the first step for an uninsured woman to receive subsidized care at no cost is to schedule an appointment in a prenatal clinic. This appointment is short and involves one task: a pregnancy test. If the test is positive and the woman decides to proceed with the pregnancy, she will begin a series of eligibility requirements to qualify for the Prenatal Care Assistance Program (PCAP), the Medicaid-funded, New York State–subsidized program that offers free prenatal care to women who meet certain income eligibility requirements, irrespective of their immigration status (New York State Department of Health 2010).[2] For their first prenatal visit following a positive pregnancy test, patients are told to allow a significant amount of time, as they will need to see a financial counselor, nutritionist, social worker, and nurse. All these appointments precede the scheduling of their first visit with a CNM or obstetrician. During their PCAP intake appointment, a great deal of the work of subjectification is begun. In this visit, and usually only in this visit, women are offered the opportunity to discuss at length their home life, migration history, family medical and social history, prior pregnancies, and more. In turn, at this visit, the patient's chart is begun, a document containing not only all the medical documentation deemed relevant to her pregnancy but also a "social work report," nutritional assessment, and notes that both describe and classify her according to certain typologies and themes.

At Manhattan Hospital, "low-risk pregnancies" are channeled automatically to CNMs. This assignment represents a reversal of trends over the last century toward medicalized models of prenatal care and childbirth. In the United States, the proportion of hospital-based births attended by obstetricians has risen relative to home-based and midwife-attended births since 1900, when only 5 percent of births occurred in hospitals and about half were midwife-attended (Feldhusen 2000; also Sargent and Bascope 1996, 222; Sargent and Stark 1989). By 1975, less than 1 percent of deliveries were midwife-attended (Centers for Disease Control 2009, 16). In 2006, however, numbers of midwife-attended births showed a rebound. While 99 percent of babies were born in hospitals and 91.5 percent of babies were delivered by an obstetrician, 7.9 percent of babies were delivered by a midwife, an eightfold increase over 1975 (Centers for Disease Control 2009, 67). Midwife-attended births have been widely shown by research to be more cost-effective and to result in fewer interventions including cesarean sections, use of epidural anesthesia, forceps delivery, and labor augmentation (Van Teijlingen, et al. 2004; Devries 2004, 311; Goer 1995; Davis-Floyd 1992, 177–184). In spite of this evidence, high malpractice premiums and an overall misunderstanding about the efficacy of midwifery care in low-risk pregnancies have led to a rapid decline in midwifery practice in the United States (Allday 2007; Epstein 2008). As a result midwifery has, for the most part, become an elite privilege for a small percentage of women of high socioeconomic and educational status who are willing to seek it out and able to pay a premium for such care (González 1986, 248–249).

Although in the United States Hispanic women are more likely than any other ethnic group except Native Americans to deliver with a midwife, the percentage of Hispanic women who do so has remained below 6 percent (Parker 1994, 1140; see Declercq 2009, 95). Yet, at Manhattan Hospital, midwife-attended prenatal care and births are the norm. It seemed to me innovative, even radical, that Manhattan made midwifery its standard of care, even though its prenatal clinic is populated largely by Medicaid recipients. I was drawn to Manhattan in large part because of this policy.[3]

Indeed, at Manhattan Hospital, I observed that, within the prenatal clinic's tracking system, those women who were placed in the midwifery section were treated to an approach to their pregnancies that was very different from the approach often described for poor minority women in the United States (Browner and Press 1996; Maraesa and Fordyce, forthcoming). Mexican patients, in particular, seemed sometimes to be temporarily exempted from the "assumption of minority" theorized by Aizita Magaña and Noreen Clark (1995), at least by their primary prenatal care providers, the midwives, and in the overall structuring of care. Within assumptions of minority dysfunction, women of color are assumed to be at greater risk than white women for health complications, and poverty itself is cast as a risk factor and proxy for certain disadvantages and behaviors. This assumption is related to Kenneth Gergen's notion of "deficit discourses," in which people are constructed according to their problems (1994). Such assumptions make little sense in light of evidence like the birth-weight paradox for Latina immigrant women. Although Manhattan does not track women into midwifery protocols because of the birth-weight paradox but rather because, overall, statistics indicate better and more economical outcomes in most low-risk pregnancies and deliveries with a midwifery approach, an epiphenomena of this tracking is a destabilization of such specious assumptions. Assumptions of minority dysfunction do seem to operate in the high-risk wing of the prenatal clinic, in interactions in labor and delivery, and with nutritionists, social workers, and other personnel. Nonetheless, the point of departure for care in this hospital seemed to me to be utterly radical in comparison with the care women described at other New York hospitals and the care scholars have described in other settings (Browner and Press 1996; Davis-Floyd and Sargent 1996; Martin 1992, 1996).[4] I describe below the experiences Mexican immigrant women recounted to me as they made their way through the prenatal clinic over the course of their pregnancies.

Getting an Appointment

Women's first interaction with the prenatal clinic is often by phone. A prospective patient or sometimes her partner, relative, or friend calls the appointments line. If it's the first few days of the month, the new appointments have just been spilled into the system, and those who call will be told they can get an appointment. If it is later in the month, they are told there are no appointments. The appointments line is for all ob-gyn services, and the number of appointments for women who do not think they are pregnant (for routine gynecological exams or other issues) is small. Women who believe they are pregnant are supposed to be given an appointment, while women who wish to schedule a gynecological appointment for any other issue may need to wait months or to seek care at another location. Often, the phone lines ring continuously throughout the day and the physician's assistants who cover them answer over and over. When there are no appointments, they sometimes seem as frustrated as the callers and are less patient with their explanations. Sometimes they explain kindly that the caller could try phoning Planned Parenthood or an affiliated hospital on the Lower East Side that seemed to have more availability or go to the emergency room. However, as the day wore on, I sometimes heard them pick up the phone over and over, repeat simply, "We have no appointments," and hang up. Here is a typical call: "There are no appointments." Then, "There are no appointments, you'll have to call back." Then, "I don't know, there are no appointments in the system." When it was late in the month, I tried to help by answering the phone. Knowing my only choice was to tell callers there were no appointments, I did not fear making a mistake. The incessant ringing of the phone and pleading of caller after caller were indeed frustrating. At one point, I asked a nurse whether she felt other hospital personnel knew how hard it was to handle the phones. She turned to me and said, "We're the front lines! They don't understand."

Once patients have obtained an appointment and come in for their first visit, they arrive at the prenatal clinic and wait in a brief queue at the registration desk. Generally, patients were treated politely. Some kinds of patient behavior, however, elicited exasperation and reprimands from the staff. Patients who arrived late—even by a few minutes—were sometimes subjected to reproach and a loud and indignant discussion of their tardiness by hospital staff. One intake employee said about—and in front of—a woman who arrived at the clinic just before 3:00 P.M., "The nerve these women have to show up at this hour and think they'll be seen!" Front-desk staff attempted to punish late patients, telling them they would not be seen or they would have to wait until everyone else was seen. I frequently saw that these threats were not carried out, as the waiting list of patients often moved quickly later in the day and patients were seen in a timely fashion. But sometimes the threats alone resulted in a patient's leaving on the spot. One young woman lowered her voice to a whisper and begged the Spanish-speaking intake clerk to do her a favor and allow her to be seen. The intake clerk responded, "Aunque yo te haga el favor, mira, no te van a ver. Aquí cerramos a las cinco, no te van a atender" [Look, even though I do you a favor, they're not going to see you. We close here at five and they are not going to see you]. The clerk put the woman's slip up on the counter, queuing her to be attended, and within ten minutes she had not only been called by a physician's assistant but had emerged and headed toward the exit with a light step. Other patient behaviors deemed unacceptable by staff included complaining about the clinic's routines or the time it took to be seen. Patients who sat patiently without complaint were typically treated politely.

Patients were asked whether they held private insurance or Medicaid. If they had neither, which was the norm for many first-time patients here, they were given a temporary identification card and told to file for PCAP. In the interim, before their PCAP enrollment was completed, new patients' personal information was entered into the system and a card was generated containing their name, address, date of birth, and "self-pay"; "self-pay" was also imprinted on all their medical documentation. If they already were enrolled in Medicaid, their identification number was stamped instead of "self-pay." I did not observe any woman who had private insurance although some women's charts continued to be stamped "self-pay" later in their pregnancies, indicating they were uninsured and also not covered by Medicaid. The physician's assistant usually then pointed at a basket of paper cups and slim plastic tubes and told the new patient, "Do your urine." I observed more than one new patient respond to this command with a quizzical expression. Whether it was because the command was given in rapid-fire speech or because the mechanics of collecting a urine sample were not familiar was not always clear. Women who were confused, asked follow-up questions, or made requests were often subject to exasperated treatment on the part of the desk attendants, who might roll their eyes, sigh, or repeat their instructions in a louder voice. Women who seemed already to know what to do were rewarded with efficient, cool respect. At the same time, it did not behoove women to seem overly familiar with the process. As the saying goes, "Familiarity breeds contempt," and women who were too well versed in the routines were sometimes looked down on as "repeat customers." Physician's assistants and others sometimes told me, "We know her already," or "This mommy has been here four times!" This dynamic was effectively described by Khiara Bridges, an anthropologist conducting research in the same clinic. She found that the clinic constructed patients as "uneducated and unintelligent, yet somehow incredibly shrewd, manipulators of the [hospital] 'system'" (2008).

Once a woman's pregnancy was confirmed, she was eligible for a PCAP Initial Prenatal Evaluation consisting of the following elements:

> Medicaid presumptive eligibility determination (completion of the Medicaid application process including the interview, assisting in the collection of documentation and forwarding the application package to the local social service district); a complete history, physical examination and pelvic examination; risk assessment including medical and psychosocial factors; laboratory screening; lead screening; prenatal genetic risk screening; initiation of patient education; screening for nutritional status; and nutrition counseling and enrollment in the Supplemental Food and Nutrition Program for Women, Infants and Children (WIC). (New York State Department of Health 2010)

Here I describe some of these steps in detail based on participant observation and interviews.

Social Work Profile

After "doing her urine," a patient's next step in the PCAP intake procedure was a visit with a social worker to produce a "psychosocial profile." I observed several PCAP intake interviews with a hospital social worker I will call Annette. She was an energetic and lively interlocutor. When I observed these interviews, I watched as women's own narratives were interrupted with the social worker's need to conform her notes to a specific format: "Wait, mami, don't tell me about that yet, just tell me who you live with." She followed a script contained on her computer screen, to which she input patient responses, but she also varied from the script in ways that seemed intended to garner increased confidence from patients.

I observed a particularly complex interview with a woman named Carmen, who was seeking to transfer from Metropolitan Hospital, discontented with the care she received there. The most seamless way to transfer would have been to request that her records be sent from Metropolitan to Manhattan Hospital, but Carmen thought she could simply move from one site to another without withdrawing her records. She informed Annette that she was given a positive HIV diagnosis at Metropolitan Hospital. She was nearly seven months pregnant, and Annette seemed to immediately engage her problem-solving skills to assess Carmen's needs as well as complete her PCAP assessment. Carmen's case is atypical in that she is the only patient I interviewed who was HIV-positive and most women in the study were involved in relationships of longer duration than hers. I include this section on a woman who was, in many ways, an "outlier" for the ways that she illustrates important dynamics in the encounter between social workers and patients, and the gendered risks of migration.

Carmen did not have proof of her HIV status, so Annette told her she might need to undergo a new test at Manhattan and also asked whether she had been given any antiretroviral medications to take. She said she had not. She said she had been given pills, but she could not tolerate them; it was not clear whether these were antiretrovirals or prenatal vitamins. She said her partner was awaiting the results of his HIV test, but because he did not have Medicaid, he was concerned he would not be able to obtain medical care if he needed it. Annette informed her that her partner could receive medications free of charge. She also said, "No tienen que dejar que la enfermedad les acabe" [You don't have to let this illness be the end of you].

Annette then went back to her script and asked Carmen about her financial and living circumstances. She had been living with her partner for four months. He and a cousin maintained her. Annette asked, "¿No coges cupones?" [You don't get food stamps?]. She said that she did not. Annette said, "Cuando nazca tu bebé, tu cualificas [sic] para cupones y asistencia si necesitas" [When your baby is born, you qualify for food stamps and assistance if you need it].[5]

Annette asked Carmen whether her pregnancy was planned, how she felt about it, and whether she had family members in the area to help her. Carmen answered that the pregnancy was somewhat planned, "Más o menos," and that her partner, who is of Venezuelan and Puerto Rican descent, was happy about the pregnancy. Annette offered her a psychological referral several times, but Carmen said that she was not depressed and that she was excited about the pregnancy: "Tenemos todas las ilusiones."

Carmen also mentioned being frustrated with the lack of care at Metropolitan, where she said no one weighed her, took her blood pressure, or told her what she needed to do given her HIV status. Annette advised her not to tell anyone she was HIV positive. She then said she would probably need a cesarean section and that she would not be able to breastfeed, to which Carmen replied, "Sí lo sé, eso es lo peor" [I know that; it's the worst part].

Carmen's interview encompassed special issues that were not typical, but each of Annette's social work summaries focused on many of the same areas, which are part of every patient's medical chart: interest level and involvement of the "FOB" (father of the baby), social and financial support, prior pregnancies, attitude and reaction about this pregnancy, history of domestic abuse and substance abuse, and so on. Although the questions were the same, the responses and the social worker's insertion of them into a semi-narrative form, which was permitted by the format she used, enabled a rich amount of information to emerge, including patient's place of birth, migration history, time in the United States, prior pregnancies, and more. At no other point during their prenatal care were women likely to be asked about their living situation or about their migration experiences.

When I spoke with Annette informally about her work, she gave me a response that belied the attentiveness and compassion I had observed in her interactions with patients. When she asked me what my research was about, I told her I was interviewing Mexican immigrant patients about their experiences in the prenatal care clinic. I asked her if she had any observations about the Mexican patients with whom she interacted. "They're a big problem," she replied. "They don't know who the father is; they have a husband and other boyfriends on the side. They don't want their husband to find out about the boyfriend." Given that this was her immediate response to my question and the morally superior tone she used, which was out of keeping with her professional role, I was taken aback. Further, her observation did not correspond in the least either to trends I had observed in my own interviews with patients or, more important, to the social work summaries she prepared, which I read at length during chart review. Of the sixty-one Mexican women patients with whom I conducted extended interviews, only four were not living with the father of their baby, a fact usually noted by the social workers. The vast majority of my interviews and Annette's own summaries described women who were in stable relationships, optimistic, and happy about their pregnancy, whether planned or not. In fact, anecdotally, many providers remarked to me that their explanations for the birth-weight paradox were the "family-centeredness," "strong social networks," and "positive attitudes about pregnancy" of Mexican immigrant patients, theories borne out by scholarly research (Hessol and Fuentes-Afflick 2000; Sherraden and Barrera 1996; Viruell-Fuentes and Schulz 2009).

I asked Annette whether she found a difference between women who had migrated recently and women who had migrated as children or were born here.

She said the behavior (multiple partners, doubts about paternity) was the same for both but that recent migrants were more fearful because they did not have many other places to go if their partner learned the baby was not his. She said evidence of this observation was the reluctance many women had to report domestic violence. "They know they'll get a worse beating. If they go straight into the shelter system from here, they are turned to homeless shelters." Annette then said confidingly, "They are sent to an intake center, where they have to talk to a social worker who is usually black and harsh with them. They immediately begin to investigate and the process is frightening to them; they're too vulnerable." I asked her whether she had observed that domestic violence lessened during pregnancy, a tendency I had heard some people describe for Mexican immigrant women. "No, they beat them anyway. They don't care. The men are nice when they come here with their wife, but at home they beat them."

Annette appeared to have preconceived notions about Mexican patients that she retained and was eager to report even though the data before her disproved them. Even Carmen's case, which on its surface described an HIV-positive woman who received intermittent care and was living in a situation that was only recently stable, was more complex than the characterization of promiscuity, abuse, and uncertain paternity Annette implied was typical for Mexican patients. Carmen migrated from Estado de México, the urban state that rings the capital city. When she left, she was a university student, majoring in biochemical industrial engineering. Her university entrance exam scores were not high enough to obtain a seat at the highly coveted and extremely competitive national university, Universidad Nacional Autónoma de México, and so she opted for a private technical college that charged her a great deal in tuition. Although she did well in laboratory work, she had a harder time with the theoretical aspects of her studies. Even though her father helped her, she said she often had to decide whether to spend her money on food, clothing, or school expenses. Finally, she decided to leave her studies and migrate.

She hired a coyote to transport her across the border. Her group was assaulted in the desert by a band of thieves who stole everything she and her companions were carrying, except for a few bills she had managed to hide in her hair. Then she was caught by border patrol and returned to Mexico. While waiting in a boarding house for another chance to cross, a dispute emerged about the deposit she had paid her smugglers. She insisted she had paid; the smugglers told her the funds had never been received. To pay off her "debt" she was forced into servitude in the household of one of the smuggler's families on the Mexican side of the border. For a month, she was kept as a captive servant.

Such abuse is so frequent that many women begin using oral contraceptives in advance of their migration in order to protect against unwanted pregnancies if they are raped on their journey (Vanderpool 2008).[6] Finally, Carmen was able to make it to New York City. She worked as a live-in domestic on Long Island, then as a cashier in a cafeteria in midtown Manhattan. There, she met her partner. After a year together, she became pregnant, and they began to live together.

The stereotypes to which Annette subscribed were little applicable to Carmen's story. Although the midwife's quotes about Mexican patients at the beginning of this section were positive and Annette's characterizations were negative, neither was empirically corroborated either in the medical records these same professionals generated or in the data gathered in this study from Mexican patients. Although certain aspects of the "assumption of minority dysfunction" have been eliminated in Manhattan Hospital's approach to prenatal care, members of the staff continued to operate with assumptions and stereotypes, both positive and negative, about the Mexican patients in their care.

A Visit to the Nutritionist

The next step in the PCAP intake procedure was a visit with a nutritionist. Part of establishing eligibility for WIC nutritional assistance is the requirement that patients be certified as "at nutritional risk." Ineligible for food stamps and other welfare benefits, undocumented immigrant patients frequently expressed a strong desire for WIC. Women were sometimes accompanied in the process of certification of eligibility by female relatives or friends who coached them on how to demonstrate eligibility. Nonetheless, the process requires women to perform their neediness and worthiness in ways that sometimes run counter both to their aspirational posture as immigrants and to the pride many women have in their caretaking abilities, including administering the family budget, cooking, and providing for their families in other ways. Compared with some of the intrusive medical aspects of their first prenatal visit, the interview with a nutritionist was rather less intimidating, even fun, and in their efforts to comply with the nutritionist's expectations they sometimes seemed to forget that the expectation was for them to demonstrate nutritional inadequacy. It also was not clear that all the patients knew they needed to demonstrate nutritional inadequacy in order to be eligible for assistance. In fact, neither the nutritionist nor the patients spoke openly to me of this process as a charade. Nonetheless, it became clear to me that in many ways it was.

Matilda was nineteen years old and the mother of one child when she visited Manhattan Hospital to begin prenatal care for her second pregnancy. Her husband was employed in building maintenance, earning \$280–\$300 per week, and they lived in a four-bedroom apartment with five other adults. The nutritionist began as she customarily did, by asking Matilda to recall what she ate over the previous twenty-four hours. Matilda said she had eaten dry cereal with milk for breakfast, and stewed chicken with rice for lunch, along with a salad composed of lettuce, carrots, and cucumber. She ate two slices of melon, two apples, and two kiwis as snacks throughout the day. For dinner, she had another bowl of cereal with milk and had drunk a soda. Over the course of a week, she was asked to estimate how often she ate different kinds of foods. For protein, she said she usually ate chicken or eggs, each two to three times per week. She did not eat red meat. She ate tortillas every day and sometimes bread in the evening, including pan dulce. She consumed fruit, fruit juices, and smoothies, and vegetables more times than she could count. When she finished this exercise, the nutritionist told her she needed to eat more vegetables, and to avoid soda, pan dulce, and sweet cereals. She showed her an image of the "food pyramid" and said, "Esto necesita todos los días" [This is what you need every day], without explaining the many ways that Matilda was already conforming with the nutritionist's expectations or signaling specific areas of concern. The overall message given to Matilda was that she was not complying with a healthy diet.

The nutritionist was born in India and conducted interviews with patients in several languages including Hindi, Urdu, and Spanish. Her Spanish was proficient, if accented and flat. Although the words she used were most often correct, her tone sometimes produced confusion. She asked questions like "¿Qué comió ayer?" [What did you eat yesterday?] in the same tone of voice as she asked, "¿Come tierra?" [Do you eat dirt?]. With questions like the latter, patients frequently leaned forward and asked her to repeat herself, as they seemed to think they had misheard. Unlike the social worker's computerized form, which allowed her to insert as much or as little detail in each field as she wished, the nutritionist's hard-copy form had little space for comments or notes. Although the twenty-four-hour recall of what women ate allowed them to speak in free form and women frequently seemed comfortable with and even to enjoy this process, describing certain foods as delicious or emphasizing foods that corresponded with what they told me in interviews were healthy diets for a pregnant women, this comfort seemed to pass as the interview continued. The nutritionist read the remainder of the questions rapidly, without prefatory comments or banter. As such, women frequently responded with single-word answers; it appeared that they attempted to keep the same pace as the nutritionist. Inevitably, at the bottom of the rear side of the form came the same condemning finding: "Diet is nutritionally inadequate."

In interviews, patients told me that at Manhattan the staff was respectful of their culture, their diet, and parenting styles, and they complained to me about the advice they had been given in other hospitals. Many women who had been diagnosed with gestational diabetes or higher than average glucose levels told me they had been advised by nutritionists in other hospitals and clinics to cut tortillas out of their diet.[7] At Manhattan Hospital, in contrast, the nutritionist displayed comprehension of Mexican patients' typical diets. She used an inductive approach in her interviews, asking women to recount what they ate; from that information she built a plan to improve the woman's nutritional intake rather than prescribing a "one size fits all" diet for all patients. I asked her whether she knew of colleagues in other institutions recommending that women with high blood-glucose levels eliminate tortillas from their diets, as I had heard. She responded that there is nothing wrong with tortillas. She said that one tortilla is an equivalent source of carbohydrates to one small potato or one piece of bread and that women could consume them as part of a balanced diet, as many as two and a half per day. Although a typical Mexican diet might include more than that, especially in lower-income households with a relative lack of other kinds of food, the nutritionist was inclined to affirm patients' habits and work to improve them. "Sometimes women do not eat a lot of meat, but they eat beans and tortillas, which is fine. It has protein."

When a woman was sent for follow-up visits with the nutritionist because of high glucose levels or rapid weight gain (or insufficient weight gain), the nutritionist sought to identify the habits of the patient that might be the cause of her problem. One patient was asked for a twenty-four-hour recall after her provider discovered that she was gaining weight too quickly. She proceeded to provide a rapid, detailed list of foods she had consumed the day before and then sat, looking expectantly at the nutritionist:

> *Nutritionist*: ¿No comió pan ayer? [Didn't you eat any bread yesterday?]
> *Patient*: Oh, sí. [Oh, yes.]
> *Nutritionist*: Y papas, ¿no comió? [And you didn't eat any potatoes?]
> *Patient*: Oh, sí, sí, comí. [Yes, yes, I ate them.]
> *Nutritionist*: Y soda, ¿tomó? [And soda, did you drink any?]
> *Patient*: Sí, sí tomé. [Yes, I drank soda.]

This slightly humorous exchange revealed that the patient had eaten far more than she had remembered initially. The nutritionist later told me that patients sometimes forget or try to hide what they have eaten for fear of getting into "trouble." She said she tells them that if their blood sugar does not improve, they will need to inject insulin. "And they don't want that. So usually they start bringing in very accurate recalls, and they tell me, 'I ate too much rice' or 'I had a piece of cake.'" The nutritionist sends patients with gestational diabetes home with a color-coded plan: red ink to indicate the times they need to check their blood, and black ink to indicate meals or snacks. She stated that they usually become adept at noting down relevant information and managing their intake.

Nonetheless, in spite of the nutritionist's constructive approach, the overall message given patients about their diets was negative. Although patients were not shown the form in their charts that read "diet needs improvement," the nutritionist also did not tell them, or me, that because her interview with them was part of an eligibility process designed to enable them to access WIC, for the encounter to be "successful," every woman who went through her office would be found "at nutritional risk" as part of that process. The PCAP procedures, in fact, explicitly state that they are conducted within an assumption of "presumptive eligibility." Although this procedure is surely more humane and results in fewer unjust denials of services than its opposite, a presumption of ineligibility, it reinforces the notion that PCAP patients are inherently needy. Further, the interviews frequently ended with advice—"No frito [sic], no soda, no pan dulce" [No fried foods, no soda, no sweet bread]—or occasionally with a more elaborate speech, such as this one, which was given to Jessy, a woman whose story will be told in detail later in this chapter:

> No pan dulce, de sal. Con lechuga y tomate. Tres comidas al día. Vegetales, frutas, todas las veces. No agua de sabor, fruta. No mucho grande [sic], vaso de jugo. Arroz al vapor, cocido en agua, no aceite. *Low-fat yogurt*. No grasa en la leche. *'Light' means* no grasa. No comida china. No frito. No azúcar. No come [sic] tarde. Camina un poco después de cena.

> [No sweet bread, only savory. With lettuce and tomato. Three meals a day. Vegetables, fruit, all the time. No flavored water, fruit. Not very big, glass of juice. Steamed rice, cooked in water, not oil. Low-fat yogurt. No fat in the milk. Light means no fat. No Chinese food. No fried [foods]. No sugar. Don't eat late. Walk a little after dinner.]

Invariably women received the message that the diet they had painstakingly narrated was not adequate. Further, they were told to abruptly and completely eliminate foods that in moderation present little or no risk to a normal pregnancy. At the same time, they were not praised for their diets, which, like Matilda's, frequently included large quantities of fresh fruits and vegetables.

Because the interview was part of an eligibility procedure, to praise women for eating well would undercut the purpose of the meeting, which was to find them nutritionally inadequate and to establish their eligibility for nutritional assistance.

Along with advice, the nutritionist distributed materials and information. Although the hospital seemed to have a low budget for patient educational materials—only a few informational sheets were routinely photocopied and given to patients over the many months they received prenatal care—the nutritionist and social worker had stacks of glossy, often bilingual, brochures provided by private corporations, including Kraft and General Mills; they liberally distributed these materials to patients. These brochures gave advice about a "healthy diet," featuring the food pyramid, and also numerous endorsements of the corporations' own products such as dry cereals, macaroni and cheese, sliced and individually packaged American cheese, and more.

In another hospital, María Pacheco's experiences with the advice of nutritionists had serious consequences. While under prenatal care for her first pregnancy at another Manhattan hospital, she was diagnosed with gestational diabetes and sent to a high-risk clinic. She was told to report there every week, where she was weighed and submitted to frequent checks of her blood glucose. She told me that she was struck by the attitude of the other women in the clinic, predominantly *morenas* and *dominicanas*, African Americans and Dominicans, who she said complained vociferously in the waiting room about the mandates given them in the clinic: "Ellas dicen que si quieren comer un pedazo de pastel, lo van a comer, que nadie les puede decir que no. Pero por mi parte, si me dicen que algo es para el bien de mi bebé, lo voy a hacer" [They say that if they want to eat a piece of cake, they're going to eat it, that no one can tell them not to. For my part, if they tell me I need to do something for the good of my child, I'm going to do it.]

On the surface, María fits a high-risk profile for low birth weight and other pregnancy complications: unmarried (although only in the legal sense), a sixth-grade education, no insurance, low-income, living in the Bronx neighborhood of Mott Haven, a neighborhood with some of the poorest health indicators in New York City (Karpati et al. 2003). However, diligence and earnestness are not measured by such health indicators, and, in spite of challenges, María was determined to do whatever her medical providers told her she needed to ensure she had a healthy pregnancy.

At the high-risk clinic, the nutritionist did not tell María the parts of her diet that were acceptable or unacceptable but instead gave her a list of foods that she should consume to maintain a healthy blood-glucose level. María went to the supermarket, list in hand, to purchase the items on the list. She told me that it was difficult to adopt such a radically new diet so quickly, but she felt it was necessary to do so. For breakfast, she had been told, she should have a half cup of cornflakes with skim milk. For a snack, a nonfat yogurt. She was told to eliminate tortillas, which she said she was told would "convertirse en azúcar" [turn into sugar.] She described standing at the stove, warming fresh corn tortillas over an open flame for her husband's meals and being nearly overcome by desire to eat one, but she said she maintained self-discipline and did not consume them. She said that sometimes she felt faint, as though she had not consumed enough nutrients to sustain her, but she assumed that she was doing the right thing by following the diet she had been given. When she returned the following week to the clinic, at her weigh-in she was told she had lost seven pounds. The doctor looked at her aghast: "Qué has hecho?" [What have you done?]. She replied to the doctor that she had followed the diet the nutritionist had given her. She told me, "Y me regañaron, me dijeron que había puesto en peligro a mi bebé. Me dijeron que no tenía que hacerlo de un solo jalón, sino de a poco. Pero nunca me dijeron eso" [And they scolded me; they told me I had endangered my baby. They said that I didn't need to do it all at once, but little by little. But they never told me that.] Although it is impossible to infer the provider's interpretations of María's rapid weight loss in the middle of her second trimester of pregnancy, it is clear that the advice she was given was not transparent. Perhaps other patients in the clinic gave the appearance of being or in fact were noncompliant with provider instructions and for that reason providers overstated the case for dietary restrictions, imagining that their guidelines would not be followed. Or perhaps providers assumed that women with low levels of formal education, such as María, would be unable to understand overly specific dietary advice, and thus it was given without thorough explanation. Irrespective of the reasons for María's being given the advice she was, by precisely following that advice, she potentially brought more risk to a pregnancy already classified as risky only to be scolded for her obedience to providers' mandates.

Further, the provider who told María she had gone too far in adapting a new diet was not the same doctor she had seen on her previous visit. Indeed she never saw the same provider twice. Ironically, continuity of care seems least available in high-risk clinics. Such clinics are often staffed by ob-gyns who dedicate one day per month to them. Consequently, patients like María never have the opportunity to "prove" themselves as compliant and capable managers of their own self-care. Instead, María's risk factors, a quick summary in her medical chart glanced at by a new doctor each week at the high-risk clinic, served as her introduction and as arbiter of the quality of care she received. Care is distributed under an assumption of risk, noncompliance, and inability to understand instructions.

Nurse and Health Educator Visits

At Manhattan Hospital, after seeing the nutritionist, the patient visits the nurse, who asks about contraception, counsels the patient about various potential pregnancy complications, and explains the trajectory of prenatal care and delivery. This information is acknowledged by the nurses to be overwhelming to many mothers in its quantity. Further, because this interview comes at the end of the long and exhausting PCAP intake process, women are often hungry and tired by the time they sit down with a nurse. Many of the topics discussed will be repeated at other visits, although women are not again given an overview of what to expect.

PCAP regulations require that women be counseled about contraception at various steps in their prenatal and postpartum care. A nurse asks in her initial PCAP intake interview, "Cómo te vas a proteger cuando tu bebé nazca?" [How are you going to protect yourself when your baby is born?] and counsels the patient about contraception. For a woman in the middle of her first prenatal appointment, this may seem an odd question. If she says she wants to have a tubal ligation, the nurse begins the paperwork for informed consent so that everything will be ready for the procedure to be performed when she delivers her baby. If she says condoms, she will be told they frequently fail and she should consider *la inyección* (Depo-Provera), or an interuterine device. If she says she has not considered contraception, she is told she must, not least because she will be asked this question a dozen more times over the course of her pregnancy and her answer will be dutifully recorded each time. Jessy was asked about contraception by a registered nurse who had called her in to discuss a diagnostic she needed to complete in the thirty-seventh week of her first pregnancy. She said that she had discussed contraception already with the health educator. The nurse insisted, and Jessy replied that she planned to use condoms. The nurse responded, "Si eso es lo que quieres, nadie te puede convencer. Tenemos la inyección, cosas más seguras" [If that's what you want, no one can convince you. We have the injection, more secure options.]

Eva was twenty weeks pregnant when I met her at the Queens immigration organization where I conducted research in 2006. I asked her how many children she had. She told me that this child would be her fifth. She had twin fourteen-year-old daughters whom she left in Mexico when she migrated. In Queens, she had given birth to two daughters, eight and five years old at the time. She said she and her partner were still trying to have a boy, but that she was not sure they would continue trying if this baby was also a girl; five is enough, she told me. She said that when she went to the hospital for prenatal care, she told the nurses she had only two children. She told me that if the hospital personnel knew this was her fifth child, they would sterilize her when the baby was born. "But, it is your choice, no?" I asked. "No, they just do it. They think we Mexicans have too many kids."[8] Karen, in contrast, came to Manhattan Hospital from Saint Vincent's, a Catholic hospital, for prenatal care with her fourth pregnancy because, she told me, she could not have obtained sterilization at Saint Vincent's. Lizbet, pregnant with her fifth child, told me that she wanted to have a tubal ligation. Like Karen, she had begun the paperwork and counseling required for the procedure.

In their twentieth week of pregnancy, prenatal patients are scheduled to meet with a childbirth educator, who has about fifteen minutes to discuss signs of impending labor, danger signs in late pregnancy, when to come to the hospital, what to expect during labor and delivery, symptoms of postpartum depression, breastfeeding, and so on. In the meetings I observed, the educator, using rapid-fire Spanish with regional colloquialisms that may not be familiar to Mexican patients, recited a lengthy script animated by her enthusiastic impressions of a laboring woman seeking a comfortable position during contractions or a mother struggling to calm a fussy baby. Every few minutes, she paused ever so briefly to say, "¿Tú entiendes, mami?" [You understand, Mommy?], and the reply was always a wide-eyed nod of the head. In spite of the frenetic pace of the presentation, the educator was always sure to mention that families need to take their babies home in a car seat, that breast milk is best (but if formula is used, do not dilute it), and parents should never, ever sleep with their baby, all American Pediatric Association guidelines that she was required to transmit.

Even as they move along this assembly line, women are living their own narratives, which sometimes facilitate the role they are cast to play as "Medicaid patients" and sometimes directly contradict it. The desire of women to qualify for the services offered under the PCAP program puts them in a bind. Their aspirations for eligibility contradict the ideas many have of themselves as "good mothers" who care for their pregnancies and provide for their children. Further, many migrants share the view that the United States offers greater access than Mexico does to the needs of life because of the higher wages available even to workers who lack formal work authorization and training (Dreby 2010; Massey and Sánchez 2010). Many women told me in interviews that in the United States one can afford what one needs. This statement applied to basic needs, like food, but also to antojos and indulgences for themselves and their children. Alma told me, "Aquí luego mi niño, lo que quiere, si se porta bien, se lo compramos, pero allá no, no se puede" [Here, if my son wants something and he behaves, we buy it for him. But there, no, one can't do that]. This assertion is related to the concept of being capable of resolving problems or troubles, or *resolver*, as described by Mexican immigrants in other contexts (Gálvez 2010). Thus, the PCAP requirement of demonstrating need in spite of what many immigrant women describe as a state of relative economic stability compared with their situation before migration is ironic and difficult to reconcile.

"I Don't Have Time for a Mommy Who Cries All Day": Negotiating Care in Labor and Delivery

It was 10:30 in the morning, July 31, 2007. Jessy called me from a taxi. She was in labor and wanted to know whether I would meet her at the hospital. A short while later, I met her on the ninth floor.[9] She had tears in her eyes and was trembling. She was alone, but her husband was on his way. She said she was worried, that water was coming out. A nurse told me to put scrubs on over my clothes and asked me who authorized me to be there. I showed her my hospital identification and said that Jessy asked me to be with her. Throughout the morning, I noticed the nurses and physician's assistants pointing at and discussing me. They seemed worried that I might be there to keep tabs on them.

The nurse, who later said she was from the Philippines, assessed Jessy:

"¿Baby mover? [sic]" [Baby move?]

"Sí" [Yes].

"¿Agua?" [Water?].

"Sí" [Yes].

A doctor came in and without introducing herself said, "No comer. Ni agua" [Don't eat or drink]. And then, "¿Pecho, bebé?" [literally, "breast, baby," but which I took to be her way of asking Jessy whether she planned to breast-feed her baby]. Even when the doctors and nurses were speaking Spanish, Jessy looked quizzically at me before answering; the monosyllabic and truncated Spanish was difficult for her to decipher. Before long, the nurses and doctors as well as Jessy looked to me to translate. A few moments later, the nurse told her that if she wanted an epidural, she should ask for it in advance because it would take time to order it and she would have to be completely still to receive it. Jessy had told me in an interview weeks earlier that she preferred not to have anesthesia: women did not need it in the past, she said; she thought it was more normal and natural to feel the pain.

Jessy migrated at the age of twenty from Achocopán, outside of Atlixco, Puebla, six years prior to our meeting at Manhattan Hospital while she was in the seventh month of her first pregnancy. She thought two children would be an appropriate number to have so that they could study the way she felt she had been unable to do. Her mother told her that she should have a big family, preferably nine children, as she had. Jessy's education stopped at the sixth grade, *la primaria*, while her husband finished middle school, *la secundaria*. He comes from a family of four sons, three of whom live in New York City.

I met Jessy in the prenatal clinic weeks before. I interviewed her on one visit, and on another I accompanied her to see the nutritionist and a nurse. She had gained twenty-nine pounds in thirty-seven weeks of pregnancy, within an average and recommended range (25–35 pounds), but was told that an abrupt increase in weight had been detected since her last visit. She said that she thought that in Mexico women were told not to gain more than one kilo per month of pregnancy, so, according to her understandings of appropriate weight gain, she thought that indeed she might have gained too much weight since her last visit. The nutritionist asked her what she ate. She said she did not think she had been eating differently but would make an effort to cut out sweets such as popsicles and ice cream, as well as fried snacks. The nutritionist noted down Jessy's plan to avoid further dramatic weight gain.

From the nutritionist, she was passed directly to a nurse who told her that perhaps the weight she had gained was due to a retention of fluids, a symptom that could be associated with various dangerous complications including toxemia, pregnancy-related hypertension, which can lead to pre-eclampsia, a disorder associated with edema and fluid retention, as well as protein in the urine. The nurse gave Jessy a jug and told her she would need to collect her urine over twenty-four hours in the jug, then return to the hospital for it to be analyzed. I was alarmed on hearing this request because ordering a diagnostic exercise such as this so late in her pregnancy was a sign of a problem that cutting back on sweets was little likely to resolve. Jessy was not given any guidance, however, about how to reconcile the conflicting advice and interpretations of her weight gain given within a few minutes' time by the nutritionist and the nurse. As we sat in the research office afterward, Jessy asked me what she should do. I asked her what she thought she should do, given the advice she had been given. She told me she would try to cut back on sweets, but that she would focus on the urine collection, as that seemed more serious. Señora Mercedes, an older Mexican woman who was assisting my research, asked her whether she drank soda. Jessy said she sometimes did, to which Mercedes replied, "Soda es un pecadote, un pecado de gula" [Soda is a big sin, a sin of gluttony].

Even though Jessy was able to proceed with her pregnancy until her labor began spontaneously, by the time she arrived at the hospital to deliver, she was prepared to consider her pregnancy as high-risk and any interventions as necessary.

Jessy's husband arrived at the hospital a short while after she did, and the nurse commanded him to stand at the head of her bed. As the day went on, Jessy's pain and discomfort increased. Even though she had seen midwives for prenatal care, as was routine at Manhattan for low-risk pregnancies, and had been classified as a good candidate for the birthing center, it was closed the day she went into labor. In fact, the birthing center was almost always closed. The midwives told me that the nurses routinely ordered it closed because of "staffing shortages," but they felt that it was because the nurses did not like the rather more labor-intensive approach to birth, in which one midwife and one nurse attend a woman throughout her labor, without anesthesia or other interventions that make patients docile. Two years later, the medical director of Manhattan closed the birthing center indefinitely, pending the resolution of conflicts among personnel about its staffing.

As Jessy's contractions increased in frequency and intensity, she tried to stand up and sway side to side on her feet. Laboring women frequently opt for moving around during labor: gravity can aid the progression of the fetus to and through the birth canal and movement can offer some relief from the pain of contractions (Davis Floyd et al. 2009). Jessy was wired to a fetal monitor that was held to her abdomen with an elastic band around her belly, but the cords were long enough that she could stand up, even while still attached to the monitor's base. Continuous fetal monitoring has become de rigueur in many hospital births, although its utility is contested (Davis Floyd et al. 2009). With fetal monitoring frequently comes a mandate that laboring women remain prostate: nurses insist that they cannot get a "good read" unless the patient lies still on her back. Jessy's pain increased when she was lying down, while her capacity to tolerate it increased notably when she stood up. She solicited my assistance in a game of deception in which she stood at the side of the bed, swaying from side to side, and I stood at the door and alerted her when someone came our way. She would then hop back onto the bed and pretend she had not moved. This went on for a couple of hours, during which her contractions increased in frequency to every two minutes. The nurses frequently came back to adjust the monitor, muttering that, from their seats at the nurses' station, they had noticed she was producing very poor reads. I told one of the medical residents that Jessy really wanted to stand up and move around a bit during contractions, and she said to me in an exasperated tone, "She must lie down! Make her lie down!"

Uncomfortable with defying the medical professionals at the institution that authorized me to be there, but feeling that my ultimate responsibility was to Jessy, I tried to enable Jessy to do what she clearly felt she needed to do, at the same time that I sought to avoid appearing as though I was overriding the requests of the nurses and doctors. Further, although I was convinced by my reading of the literature that continuous fetal monitoring is unnecessary in most instances of labor, I was conflicted about enabling Jessy to defy its use while her medical providers were insisting it was necessary. At one point, the nurse asked Jessy how much pain she felt, on a scale of one to ten. Jessy said eight. The nurse went on to ask me whether Jessy was Mexican. I told her she was, to which the nurse replied, "It doesn't seem like she's Mexican," and told me that typically Mexican patients are good candidates for the birthing center, citing that they are very stoic, with a high pain threshold. She said to me in English, "This patient is acting as though she has a lot of pain, but her tummy is not contracting hard. Usually when they cry, it means the baby is here." A few moments later, in an attempt to make small talk, I asked the nurse whether the babies were her favorite part of her job; she answered, "Yes, they cry, but it's ok. I don't have time for a mommy who cries all day." While we talked, Jessy excused herself and spent nearly a quarter of an hour in the bathroom. The doctor came in during that interval and the nurse said, "I can't monitor her; she keeps moving around. I can't get a good read."

Jessy's contractions were not "registering" for the nurses because she was disrupting their measurement with the fetal monitor: without technological measurement of their severity, the contractions did not exist. The nurse praised Mexican patients as stoic with a high pain threshold, but the way she did it denigrated Jessy for failing to live up to that ideal. Crying and insisting on standing and moving around during labor, Jessy was perceived to be feigning: her contractions could not be strong if they were not appearing on the monitor as strong. Actually, there is no objective measure of a contraction's strength, much less of a woman's subjective experience of them. The fetal monitor only measures contractions and the space between contractions relative to each other. If a fetal monitor is interrupted and placed again, the measurements from one session are not comparable to another; contractions from early labor do not appear to be any stronger than contractions from advanced labor if the monitor has been reset. Jessy's refusal to comply with the restrictions posed by the monitoring equipment disqualified her embodied experience of labor as irrelevant and, worse, exaggerated.

While alone in the room with Jessy and her husband, he said to me, "A veces los doctores atienden bien pero regañan a uno" [Sometimes the doctors

do a good job, but they scold you]. In his statement, there was an implicit critique of the treatment his wife had been receiving at the same time that he cast
it as a price to be paid for a doctor who does a good job. Roberto Castro writes
about the scolding of women by nurses, doctors, mothers-in-law, and husbands
as a sign of the gendered inequality of reproductive health encounters in
Mexico. He notes that it is the prerogative of persons in authority to scold,
regañar, and that scolding is thus evidence of a hierarchical vision of social
relations (2002, 362). Although the public health care system in the United
States is a site of socialization of immigrant patients, patients frequently arrive
already socialized into the hierarchical social relations that characterize modern
biomedical practices. Such socialization is a function, too, of what Robbie
Davis-Floyd (1992) calls technocratic models of perinatal care and of the supplantation of other ways of knowing by authoritative knowledge, as described
by Brigitte Jordan: "To legitimize one kind of knowing devalues, often totally
dismisses, all other ways of knowing, [so that] those who espouse alternative
knowledge systems are often seen as backward, ignorant or naïve troublemakers"
(Jordan 1992, 2, quoted in Davis-Floyd and Davis 1996, 258).

A few moments later, at 3 P.M., a resident came in and proceeded to manually examine Jessy's cervix for dilation without asking permission or explaining what she was going to do. She pronounced that she was 4.5 centimeters
dilated and told her, "Mami, necesita epidural" [Mommy, you need an epidural].
Far from being given the option—in an informed-consent procedure—of chemical pain management, Jessy was given a clear mandate. The resident then told
her she had another six to eight hours of labor. Jessy assented to the epidural,
then asked me if she would still feel pain. I told her she probably would not.
"Informed consent" took the form of her signature a while later on a stack of
papers that no one explained or translated. This was the anticlimactic moment
when Jessy legally ceded control of her birth experience.

A midwife who was attending other patients that day told me in the staff
lounge that a patient who qualifies for the birth center can follow birth-center
protocol even if the patient is in regular labor and delivery and remarked that
such a protocol includes the ability to move around, without monitoring. I did
not ask these questions with direct reference to Jessy's experience, but in a
hypothetical fashion. However, even if I had asked them with the intent of
soliciting the midwife's assistance in making Jessy's care align with the
birth-center protocol she had anticipated, Jessy's placement in the care of the
obstetrical staff when she was triaged on arrival meant that she was now out
of the midwives' jurisdiction. The midwives were significantly outnumbered by
ob-gyn residents on the floor of labor and delivery, and as such delivered only

about a fifth of the babies during the period I conducted research. Birth-center-oriented options—such as the ability to move around, abstention from continuous fetal monitoring, permission to drink water or eat during labor, and alternatives to pain medication—were not offered to Jessy (Davis-Floyd et al. 2009). Had Jessy arrived at a different time or day, she might have been attended by this or another midwife.

A midwife I interviewed later, and to whom I recounted, without identifying Jessy, the insistence of the nurses and residents that she lie down told me, "Patients with doctors don't ambulate. It's just not [the doctors'] style." She said that continuous fetal monitoring not only was considered clinically important to ob-gyns but was a consequence of budget problems. She said so few nurses were put in charge of laboring patients that they relied on technology to monitor the progress of more laboring patients than they could personally attend to. She said that although the nurses were unable to attend to patients' "needs and desires," they also could not compromise medical care, so they opted for patients to remain prostate and continuously monitored.

While her husband and I waited with Jessy for the epidural she was now anxious to receive, her contractions became stronger. At one point, when a contraction came, and Jessy threw off the sheet that covered her, the nurse said, in English, "Why you not covered? You pushing?" Her husband was becoming more proactive in his assistance: he anticipated the pain of the contractions by the look on Jessy's face and massaged her lower back. Then, a resident came in and tried to get a sonogram of the baby. The resident seemed inexperienced with this kind of exam, and as she placed the wand over and over, she said to herself, "No, that's not it." Jessy became increasingly worried, her eyes darting from the monitor, to the wand on her belly, to the resident's face, to her husband, and to me. I told her that the doctor seemed to be having a problem with the machine; it was not a problem with the baby. An attending physician came in and told the resident to "give up" and "go see the patient with the forceps delivery." She also told the resident she could do a cervical exam on another patient; the resident said, "Oh, great!" and walked out smiling without a word to or glance at Jessy.

Jessy did not receive her epidural until five in the afternoon, two hours after it was ordered. Her labor was augmented with Pitocin at seven in the evening, and her baby was finally born vaginally at 1:41 in the morning. It seems clear that what might have been an uneventful and uncomplicated labor was managed by the doctors and nurses in a way that slowed its progress, increased the level of pain and discomfort felt by Jessy, and protracted the baby's birth. Although Jessy was happy with the final result, a healthy six-pound, twelve-ounce baby boy, she was disturbed by the way her labor and delivery seemed to become complicated when it had begun without complications. Jessy's chart indicated that her delivery was labeled "NSVD," Normal Spontaneous Vaginal Delivery. An increase in the frequency of interventions during labor and delivery, like the epidural and Pitocin Jessy received, normalize those interventions so that they no longer are interpreted as extraordinary. For Mexican patients I interviewed, "normal" meant vaginal but also referred to a birth without epidural anesthesia, labor augmentation, induction, forceps, and other increasingly routine interventions. Yet, "NSVD" can be far from such a vision of "normal." For Jessy's providers, it seemed in my observation of their interactions with her in labor and delivery, her labor was unusual only perhaps in her failure to behave like Mexican patients were expected to behave: her defiance of their orders to stay prostate to facilitate continuous fetal monitoring set her apart from their expectations of the stoic, docile Mexican mother. The augmentation of her labor and use of epidural anesthesia were not remarkable, their routine nature corroborated in the ways that these interventions were posed to Jessy as "necessary" and to which she had no reason to object.

Another patient, Verónica, felt that the pain she experienced in her first delivery was worsened by the mandate that she stay in a reclining position. She said that although a Puerto Rican nurse, "una Boricua," was compassionate and helpful to her, she rebelled against the instructions she was given:

> Ella me decía no, pues, tienes que aguantarte . . . no, pero, como yo me ponía, este, no sé me daba como coraje, me ponía rebelde. Yo creo por el dolor. Me decían, "haz una cosa" y yo hacía la otra porque quería quitarme ese dolor. Ella me dijo "no, no, no, tranquila," dice que, "si te paras por ahí y caminas te va a hacer mal."

> [She told me you have to withstand it . . . no, but I, it was like I became, I don't know, I became angry, I became rebellious. I think it was because of the pain. They told me, "Do this," and I did the opposite because I wanted to get rid of that pain. She told me, "No, no, no, calm down," saying, "If you stand up and you walk around it's going to cause you harm."]

> *Alyshia*: ¿Qué, le decían que tenía que estar acostada? [What, they told you you had to lie down?]
> *Verónica*: Acostada solamente querían que así estuviera, que no me sentara de la cama ni que me parara. [They wanted me lying down; they wanted me not to sit on the bed or stand up].

Alyshia: ¡Oh! Pero así se siente más el dolor, acostada [Oh! But one feels more pain lying down].

Verónica: ¡Uy! Sí, yo le decía quiero caminar para que se me quite. Pero como me tenían con tanta cosa no podía pararme. Sí. Yo no sé mucho . . . dicen que porque por la primera, primer hijo uno, este, algunas . . . es más difícil, pero dicen que los demás ya no. [Oh, yes, I said I want to walk so that [the pain] would pass. But since they had me tied up with so many things, I couldn't stand up. Yes. I don't know much . . . but they say that when it is one's first labor, first baby, for some it's more difficult, but then that with later pregnancies it's not bad].

Verónica describes what she felt as an instinct that to stand up and walk around would aid her tolerance of the pain of labor. Even though the Puerto Rican nurse is the member of her medical team whom she describes as being most compassionate (and Spanish-speaking), it is the nurse who delivers the firm mandate that Verónica will cause harm if she insists on getting up.[10] Verónica also implies that, like Jessy, she might have been inclined simply to defy the mandate if she had not been tied up with so many apparatuses. She notes that she "doesn't know much," attributing the disconnect between her own impulse and her caregivers' mandate to remain prostate as a result of her own ignorance, and she also expressed her understanding that first-time mothers experience more difficult labor, even while she asserts her own sense of how even her first labor might have been less uncomfortable had she been allowed to move around.

Esther is another woman I visited during labor at Manhattan Hospital. Thirty-four years of age, she migrated from Acatlán de Osorio ten years before. She was sent to the labor and delivery floor at ten in the morning from the prenatal clinic because she was past her estimated due date. She was induced with Pitocin while a sterile balloon was introduced into the cervix, inflated two centimeters, then pulled out to dilate the cervix. By 11:30 A.M., she was experiencing contractions that she felt strongly in spite of epidural anesthesia. While she labored, the nurse in the room, who told me she was Chinese, chatted with me, openly telling me about the patient's progress.

At three in the afternoon, when I returned to check on Esther, she and the bed she had been lying on were gone, the room empty, except for Esther's husband, standing in purple scrubs and surgical mask, and her aunt, who was sitting in a chair, holding her purse, and looking content. A nurse walked in and said, "Papi, come." She proceeded to stand close to him and adjust his hat, his sleeves, his waistband. She tucked his clothing under the scrubs and finally told him to pinch the mask at the bridge of his nose. He was nervous and she repeated each of her instructions twice, but she was patient, even tender, with the expectant father. Then, she whisked him off to surgery. "¿Qué pasó?" I asked the aunt. She told me that her niece had reached seven centimeters, "y no abrió más" [and she didn't open any more.] Doctors decided Esther needed a cesarean section. The aunt told me she had delivered her three children via cesarean sections and that it was not a big problem, especially when one has faith in God, as she assured me she did.

In both Esther's and Jessy's deliveries, the women experienced a high level of medical intervention after anticipating uncomplicated deliveries. Although I do not have the clinical expertise to question the necessity of the successive interventions experienced by these two patients, their experiences are illustrative of the complicated ways that childbirth can be shaped not only by medical protocols that are heavily oriented toward intervention but also by the attitudes and expectations of providers, laboring women, and their family members. Although Jessy thought she would deliver her baby without anesthesia, the reality of laboring while attached to sensors and cables, unable to move about or engage in pain-relieving postures and movements, progressively lowered her tolerance of pain and made her amenable to epidural anesthesia and other interventions. At the same time, her partner discussed reprimands by providers as a price one must pay for medical care. She was also given the message that her experience of pain was exaggerated and her cultural status was even brought into question: as a Mexican, she was expected to be stoic. Further, the assertion of providers that interventions were not optional, "Mami, necesita epidural," reinforced the idea that resistance, should she still have the energy for it, was futile.

Esther also labored under assumptions that her birth and postpartum recovery would resemble in some ways that of her female kin in her hometown. However, with her labor induced, augmented, anesthetized, and ultimately brought to a halt for surgery, her expectations were off the mark. Although the nurse attending her did not engage in commentary about Esther's attitudes or pain threshold, neither was the patient given an explanation for what caused her labor to go off course, except for the generic explanation noted in her chart, "failure to progress." Further, her aunt's contentment with Esther's cesarean section and assertion that religious faith mitigated the risks associated with surgery sent Esther a message about the acceptability of such interventions.

Postpartum Care

All nine of Verónica's siblings reside in New York City. Her seven sisters had their children in Izúcar de Matamoros, Puebla, prior to migrating. When

Verónica had her babies in New York City, she hoped to maintain la cuarentena, as she recalled her mother doing. "Allá, no se paran de la cama para
nada" [There, they don't get out of bed for anything]. However, she said her
hopes were thwarted because her siblings and partner work all day, and no one
could help her if she tried to stay in bed. Rubi was relatively fortunate, however, because her husband hired *una muchacha*, a young woman, for several
weeks to help her keep la cuarentena in her Brooklyn apartment while he
worked.[11] Similarly, Francisca said that, after her first delivery, her husband
and an older female acquaintance helped her guardar reposo. After the birth of
her second child, she had to get out of bed to prepare food, but her husband did
all the other *quehaceres*, chores, around the house. Similarly, Georgina told me
that she managed to partially keep la cuarentena, resting for two weeks after
birth with help from her husband and a sister, but then she had to get back to
her routine. She also said she might have liked to take an herbal steam bath, but
"no sé hacerlo de las hierbas, no tengo a mi mamá aquí" [I don't know how to
do the thing with the herbs; I don't have my mother here.]

Alma said that when she had her first child, in Morelos state, her mother-
in-law insisted she keep la cuarentena. In New York, with her second child, her
sister quit working in order to take care of her after she came home from the
hospital. She said she tried to get out of bed to help, but her sister scolded her,
telling her that she was there to cook and clean for her so she would not need
to get out of bed. Unfortunately, however, she quickly found herself back in the
hospital. She told me the baby had bruises from a forceps delivery and developed a fever leading him to be kept in the hospital for a week. She tried to
spend most of each day at the hospital with him, but because of worry, exhaus-
tion, and the long subway rides between Manhattan and her home in Queens,
she was debilitated to such a degree that she fainted and experienced a seizure
at her baby's bedside. She was kept in the hospital for tests. Ultimately, she was
told she had suffered an epileptic seizure and prescribed medication. She
contrasted her first and second pregnancies. In Mexico, she delivered her first
child at the home of a midwife. Her first son weighed more than eight pounds.
With her second child, her labor was induced and her baby was born three
weeks early at 4 pounds, 6 ounces:

> Sí, por eso, este, luego cuando platico con mi mamá le digo allá con la
> partera no quería yo ir, pero aquí tantos doctores que me echaron mon-
> tón y solo lastimaron a mi bebé. Todo fue muy triste y por eso ya no
> quiero tener otro bebé porque siento que voy a pasar por lo mismo, por
> eso no.

[Yes, for that reason, when I talk to my mother, I say, there, I didn't want to be seen by a midwife. But here, with loads of doctors working on me, all that happened was that my baby was injured. It was all very sad, and that is why I do not want to have another baby, because I feel like I'll go through the same experience. That's why.]

During Esther's labor (described above), I chatted with her husband and her aunt about their expectations for the postpartum period. Esther told me that her aunt was going to help her keep la cuarentena, but the aunt told me it might be difficult because she lived in Brooklyn, and Esther in the Bronx. The aunt told me that it was a practice common in Mexico, not New York. She said the same about baths with herbs. "Eso se llama el temazcal, pero se hace en México, acá, no" [That's called a *temazcal,* but it's done in Mexico, not here.] This, even while Esther's husband told us that in Ecuador there are similar practices of bathing a woman at five and twelve days postpartum with water boiled with *monte y vegetales,* medicinal plants and herbs. Thus, despite her husband's likely support for her desire for cuarentena and steam baths, given their similarity to practices with which he was familiar in his native Ecuador, her aunt let her know that, in her opinion, such practices were ill-suited to New York. This was similar to a conversation I had with another woman, Jacqueline, and her aunt in the recovery room after her delivery. Jacqueline gave me a great deal of information about the use of herbal remedies for all kinds of ailments, including those for postpartum healing, but her aunt said she did not think they were necessary. The aunt told me that because she had her babies in New York, she was accustomed to U.S. practices and thus preferred not to use special foods or herbs for healing after childbirth.

The subjectification that immigrant patients experience during labor and delivery continues in the postpartum period. In interviews during her pregnancy, Diana told me her sad tale of thwarted aspirations. She told me she had come from her hometown, Tetela del Volcán, in the state of Morelos *para conocer*, to get to know New York, a year and a half earlier. When she decided to stay, she had hoped she could achieve financial stability and independence. She lived with cousins and friends in Queens. She became pregnant after a short relationship, and the man disappeared after she informed him of her pregnancy. She worked caring for a friend's daughter while the friend worked in a nail salon in Manhattan. Diana earned $100 per week for eight hours of work per day, six days per week, but was charged $80 per week in rent by her housemates. When I asked her to tell me her greatest concerns about her pregnancy, she told me that she was worried about being able to provide for her child and that she felt sad about being alone. She hoped her housemates would be able to help her with basic needs until she could get back to work. I accompanied her to a follow-up visit with the social worker, Annette. Given the lack of "FOB support" noted in Diana's chart and notations about her slim resources for caring for her child, she was scheduled for more than the usual number of visits with the social worker, although she had yet to receive any tangible benefit from these visits beyond the standard allotment of groceries she received from WIC. I asked her if it was all right for me to mention her concerns about being able to provide for her baby to see whether Annette could offer additional services to her. Diana said that would be fine. Annette asked her what she felt she needed, and Diana said "everything." She said she had heard that she needed certain things for the baby but did not know what exactly or how she would be able to afford them. Annette said the infant would qualify for food stamps, but that, except for WIC, there were few benefits for which Diana, an undocumented immigrant, was eligible while pregnant.

In this conversation, it became clear that Diana would need a crib and car seat for her infant in order to bring her baby home from the hospital and also to avoid scrutiny from the Administration for Child Services (ACS). It is New York State law that newborn infants may be discharged only in a car seat. Parents who do not own a car and have plans to take their baby home on public transportation (or on foot, as in the case of some of the women I met in Queens) still needed to show a car seat in order to be discharged from the hospital.[12]

Possession and use of a crib is a less formal requirement that can still have tremendous stakes. The childbirth educator and social workers at Manhattan told pregnant women what the federal guidelines for prevention of Sudden Infant Death Syndrome required them to: that a crib is the safest place for an infant to sleep (Eunice Kennedy Shriver National Institute of Child Health and Human Development 2005). But Mexican women often co-sleep with their infants, as do women in many other places throughout the world (Davis-Floyd et al. 2009; Kimmel 2002). Studies on co-sleeping show it to be equally if not more safe than for an infant to sleep alone in a crib, in addition to offering continuity of breastfeeding and the affective benefits of mother-child bonding (McKenna 2002). Nonetheless, the American Academy of Pediatrics, even while citing studies showing that co-sleeping can be safe, recommends that infants sleep in a crib in their parents' bedroom for the first six months (American Academy of Pediatrics 2005). Many women told me co-sleeping enabled their babies to nurse without disturbing other family members and housemates and enabled them to keep certain aspects of the cuarentena (avoidance of sexual intercourse, breastfeeding, and maximal rest for the mother). They also said it was practical, as many women shared a bedroom with their immediate family members in apartments shared with other families, leaving little room for a crib.

I asked Annette whether Diana was eligible for help in getting a crib. Annette gave her a list of phone numbers associated with Catholic Charities but shrugged her shoulders when I asked whether any of them were more reliable sources for assistance than others. I offered to help Diana contact them. I called nearly a dozen numbers, but the few that answered did not serve women who were not citizens or legal permanent residents; required documentation of income and living arrangements that rivaled Medicaid eligibility processes in extent; or required families to travel long distances and attend multiple screening appointments, an impossibility given Diana's precarious employment situation. When I called Catholic Charities, I asked for someone who spoke Spanish so that I could pass Diana the phone but was transferred three times before being told that the Spanish-speaking social worker was at lunch. I was told Diana could attend a childbirth-education course to become eligible for a crib, but she would need to fill out an application and show several required documents: photo identification, proof of residence, marriage certificate, and a referral letter on hospital letterhead. The crib would be delivered after the baby was born. I eventually did make an appointment for Diana with another agency that seemed to have the most feasible requirements and encouraged her to bring her young charge with her to the appointment to avoid taking a day from work.[13]

Why would Diana need to go to such great lengths to obtain a crib, a piece of furniture commonly considered unnecessary by other Mexican mothers? Diana learned that her fragile economic status and the absence of the fetus's father and his support made her eligible for increased scrutiny on the part of state agencies. In fact, Annette told her that if a social worker paid a visit to her apartment after the baby was born and did not see a crib, she could "have problems."

I witnessed other women being told the same. I never heard a patient tell the social workers or health educators that they planned to co-sleep; the most common response to these warnings was silence. Visits to women involved in this study recruited outside of Manhattan Hospital revealed that although some families used a crib, more often than not infants co-slept with their parents. María Jacobo was pregnant with her sixth child when I visited her at her South Bronx apartment. She asked me to help her talk with a social worker who was attempting to close her case, which would mean loss of the food stamps on which she relied to feed her children. She had dispatched her husband, who was employed selling flowers outside a deli but had the day off, to do laundry down the block because, she said, if the social worker saw that her husband was involved in her life and employed, she could lose her benefits indefinitely. Her toddler, about eighteen months at the time, slept in a crib in the room she shared with her husband and two other children (the others lived in Guerrero state). Apart from the crib, the room contained a double bed and two small "toddler beds." The crib in which her toddler snored doubled as a storage space; linens and bags of disposable diapers were piled around him. The newborn she was expecting would sleep between his parents.

Of course, in spite of American Academy of Pediatrics warnings, most families are not subject to investigation of their sleeping arrangements, nor is there a law regarding such habits as there is with car seats. Nonetheless, consumption of public services and sometimes efforts to demand rights to which they are legally entitled (such as housing repairs to correct dangerous conditions) expose immigrant families to heightened scrutiny by state agencies. When María Pacheco's daughter was a baby, she shared a bed with her parents. When she was three, the couple turned a wide hallway into a second bedroom, furnished with a toddler bed and brightly colored floor mats that made it look like an appealing, if miniature, bedroom just for Jane. When her second child was born, he slept in his parents' bed and then later in a crib along the side of their bed. One night, the family was visited by a social worker at 10:00 P.M., after the landlord reported them for "child endangerment" following their removal of a window guard during installation of an air conditioner. They were involved in a dispute in housing court at the time because of the landlord's refusal to make necessary repairs to a boiler that emitted exhaust and had caused their son to experience respiratory difficulties. María interpreted the landlord's report as an effort to intimidate them into moving. The social worker, on being admitted to the apartment, demanded to know where the children were sleeping, went to their rooms, and tore off their covers. The children, ages two and eight at the time, awoke, crying and frightened. María and her husband were obliged to schedule a follow-up appointment the following day at which the children were required to be present, even though it was a school day. At that appointment, the social worker quizzed the children individually about their sleeping arrangements and asked them other questions.

Fear of ACS emerged as a recurring theme in this and in a previous research project (Gálvez 2009), even though it was not a theme I addressed in interview schedules. Families told me they nervously adjusted their parenting practices based on what they understood to be the law, telling me that they understood it to be illegal for parents to lay a hand on children and that children could always report their parents to authorities. A colleague, immigration scholar Robert Smith, told me the story of a family for whom he was advocating. The wife called 911 to report her husband, who had come home from a drinking binge and become violent. She intended to "teach him a lesson," but he was arrested and was eligible for deportation. Her children, including a breastfeeding newborn, were taken from her and put in foster care while social workers investigated signs of what they interpreted to be potential physical abuse (at the hands of the husband) and neglect. Neglect was inferred from the lack of baby food jars in the cupboard and of a crib in the bedroom. The distraught mother, having done what she thought she was supposed to do—report domestic violence—was engaged in a desperate effort to reunite her family. Stories like these abounded in conversations with immigrant mothers. Although many women said they did not personally know people who had lost custody of their children, talk of calling 911 on violent husbands, children being taken into foster care, wives being threatened with a call to *la migra*, immigration authorities, and other tales of intervention in families by state agencies were common and chilling. In their study, Jocelyn Solís, Genoveva García, and Silvana Bonil found that undocumented immigrant women were less likely than other victims of domestic violence to file a report and more likely to seek solutions to abusive situations that enabled the perpetuation of family unity (2002).

The issue of baby food in the anecdote above is illustrative of notions about food and pregnancy discussed elsewhere in this book. I have sat on a park bench, struggling with my own baby's food jar, bib, and other gear, watching a Mexican mother remove one strip of peel from a banana, and, deftly, using a spoon and the remainder of the intact banana peel as a bowl, scoop and simultaneously mash tiny bits of banana that she fed to her baby. María Jacobo sat with me at her kitchen table, feeding small bits of chicken stewed with spicy chiles to her eager toddler as he sat on her lap. Absence of baby food jars is far from a reliable indicator of absence of concern for a baby's diet. Traveling for research with my own nearly one-year-old son in Mexico City, Estado de México, and Puebla, I was offered a great deal of advice and tips about what I should and should not feed him; this advice centered largely on enabling him to eat what many Mexicans consider real food: home-cooked, flavorful fare modified for young eaters only in the size of the bites and the texture. In direct interactions with ACS and the urban legends that circulate regarding it, women are given the message that jarred baby food is the only appropriate food for infants.

With help from the friend who employed her and from private donations, Diana obtained the clothing and diapers she needed for her newborn. We were in touch shortly after he was born, and I visited her at her home in Queens. It was a neat and quiet apartment in a two-story, two-family home. She kept the door of her bedroom closed but indicated that she slept there with her newborn son. Her housemates slept in other rooms. She seemed calmer and more content than when I talked with her at the hospital, but she was not free of the heightened scrutiny that had accompanied her during her prenatal care. She showed me that the baby had a slightly protruding, soft bulge on one side of his head, without bruising or discoloration of the skin. She asked me what I thought it was—I said I did not know—and said she planned to take him to Manhattan Hospital to have it checked. When I called her a few days later, she told me they had run several tests on the infant, including an x-ray, and told her she had nothing to worry about. I asked her what they told her it was, and she said they had not given her a diagnosis. With Diana's permission, and my institutional approval to review charts, I looked up her son's charts the next time I was in the hospital. In the medical record, it was clear that her visit to the emergency room was treated as a potential abuse case. There was no indication of any possible medical causes for the lump, although the x-ray was noted not to have indicated injury. For the hospital her visit to the emergency room had as its primary purpose not the diagnosis of the abnormal bulge on her son's head, which was Diana's objective, but the ruling out of abuse. The doctor and a social worker who interviewed Diana concluded that the "baby's mother" cared for her son and could not recall doing anything that would cause a head injury. She was given guidance regarding "shaken baby syndrome" and sent on her way. Diana did not tell me that her visit was a social work intervention more than a medical one, and I, in turn, did not tell her what I saw in the chart. Nonetheless, the notations in her Manhattan chart will likely continue to follow her, and her efforts to seek medical care for her child as he grows will likely be hampered by preexisting suspicions about her capacity to properly care for him.

Immigrant Care as Socialization

Biomedical approaches to pregnancy and childbirth are ostensibly a techno-scientific response to an arena of human experience that has historically been considered both mundane and "natural" as well as "mysterious" and "unpredictable." Although the uncertainty of pregnancy and childbirth has been, in some cultures, dealt with through recourse to metaphysical practices of prayer, ritual, magic, and traditional healing methods, in Western industrialized societies it has been increasingly assigned to the realm of medical intervention. Ironically, prenatal care as routinely practiced in the United States has been demonstrated to have little to no impact on the major complications affecting birth outcomes. In his provocative book, *Expecting Trouble* (which a Manhattan Hospital midwife recommended to me), obstetrician Thomas Strong argues: "The perception that contemporary American prenatal care is an essential, unequivocally valuable commodity for our mothers persists because too few of us are capable of discerning good intentions from genuine medical knowledge. Almost one hundred years after its advent, it's still a mystery as to what actually constitutes prenatal care, nor do we know which aspects of prenatal care really confer benefit to our mothers" (2000, 6). Strong continues, "The conventional wisdom that prenatal care is crucial to the well-being of mothers and their babies is incongruent with the findings of published medical research and our nation's experience over the last half-century" (29). Dalton Conley, Kate Strully, and Neil Bennet similarly cite studies that show that prenatal care does not have a uniform impact on outcomes for women of different racial and socioeconomic categories (2003, 71). Strong argues that prenatal care, as it currently exists in the United States, is essentially a ritual through which mothers and their care providers reassure themselves that they are doing everything they can to ensure a healthy pregnancy; they perform this ritual with faith but without a great deal of evidence that it will result in the outcome they seek.

Nonetheless, as thoroughly established by anthropologists of reproduction, biomedicalized prenatal care is cast as authoritative knowledge (Davis-Floyd and Sargent 1996; Jordan 1997). Through a process of distancing pregnant and laboring women from the embodied experiences of pregnancy and childbirth, "prenatal care can be seen as a process of medical socialization, in which providers attempt to teach pregnant women their own interpretations of the signs and symptoms that women will experience as the pregnancy proceeds and the significance that should be attached to them" (Browner and Press 1996, 144).

Prenatal care is for women in the United States in general an experience of socialization into the norms, attitudes, and expectations appropriate to the pre- and perinatal period, but for immigrants this care is more fraught and complicated. The prenatal clinic is a site for medical socialization as well as immigrant assimilation. In the waiting area, exam rooms, and labor and delivery ward of Manhattan Hospital, not only are Mexican immigrant women taught how to be competent consumers of public prenatal care, but they take it as an opportunity to learn what is expected of them as mothers and citizens in the United States generally. The prenatal clinic is a site of subjectification, or subject-making, what Aihwa Ong calls "self-making and being-made by power relations that produce consent through schemes of surveillance, discipline, control and administration" (1996, 737). In turn, the providers take their interactions with Mexican immigrant patients as an opportunity both to school those patients into what is expected of them and also—positively and negatively—to compare and contrast them with others: with other immigrant and minority women and with women who are insured and native-born (see also Piven and Cloward 1971).

Public prenatal clinics, even ones as progressive as Manhattan Hospital's, are organized hierarchically. Doctors oversee the clinic, labor and delivery, the entire midwifery practice, and the birthing center. Doctors and midwives oversee nurses and physicians' assistants. Patients are referred to as consumers, but are, especially because this is a public hospital, at the bottom of the hierarchy, eligible to receive instructions, advice, and reprimands from everyone above them. Immigrant patients, Medicaid recipients, and patients with limited English are subject even to the authority of other patients, who frequently school them in ways to avoid difficulties in accessing services and care. In this way, authoritative knowledge, which is already monopolized by the figures of authority, especially doctors, is reinforced, expanded, and reproduced in ways that serve to not only decenter and displace but actually demote the other kinds of knowledge with which women arrive at the hospital.

Chapter 5

Critical Perspectives on Prenatal Care

Rosa migrated from Puebla's state capital three years prior to becoming pregnant and seeking prenatal care at Manhattan Hospital. I asked her whether she planned to have anesthesia during labor and delivery. While her husband massaged her back, she told me she did not.

> *Alyshia*: ¿Y anestesia por qué no quiere? [And why don't you want anesthesia?]
>
> *Rosa*: No sé, me gustaría sentir a mi bebé. Pienso que para eso se arriesga uno a tener bebes. Si no, ¿qué . . . qué chiste? [I don't know; I'd like to feel my baby. I think that it is the reason that one risks having babies. If not, what's the point?]

In this interchange, Rosa reveals a common view of the participants in this study. Most women interviewed expressed a disinclination toward using pain medication during labor, as well as a generally negative view about the use of medications during pregnancy and the imposition of common interventions during delivery, including cesarean section.

Even though Mexican patients are praised by providers for their purported stoicism and docility during pregnancy and labor, I found that in fact many had pronounced contrarian views about some of the protocols of prenatal care and labor and delivery that are routine in contemporary biomedical settings. In these perspectives we can see that although many of the women in the study eagerly embraced the prenatal care they received, viewing it as more modern, humane, and advanced than the care they might have been able to access in Mexico, they did not unquestioningly consume prenatal care but actively rejected some central components of it. The aspects of care that many women critiqued and rejected reveal certain commonly held ideas about pregnancy and an agentive approach to health care consumption.

There were key areas of contention between the biomedical model of care provided in Manhattan Hospital's clinic and the norms and expectations of many Mexican immigrant women. The rejection of certain aspects of care was less pronounced with greater duration in the United States. This chapter offers a corrective to the correlation proposed so far in this book, in which immigrants' aspirational stance makes them more likely than not to embrace dominant models of prenatal care in New York City's public hospitals. The data in this chapter indicate that even though Mexican immigrant women are enthusiastic about accessing what they view as a modern and technologically well-equipped hospital, that entrance into this mode of care does not erase their deeply rooted understandings of pregnancy and childbirth as tasks they were born to accomplish successfully. On the contrary, their epistemologies of pregnancy indicate that they negotiate the care they receive in the hospital with certain suppositions about their own abilities to have a healthy pregnancy and successful labor and delivery. These suppositions may be protective and part of the explanation for the birth-weight paradox. Nonetheless, they complicate the relationship between Mexican immigrant women and their prenatal care providers.

The areas of contention include attitudes about pregnancy and prenatal care in general, ideas about a healthy diet, views on chemical pain relief and the consumption of medicines during pregnancy and childbirth, and opinions about cesarean section and other increasingly routine interventions during delivery.

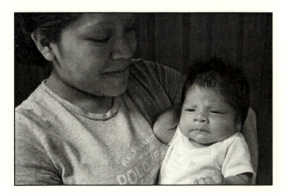

Figure 5   Proud mother with her newborn son, October 2007. Photo by the author.

Attitudes about Pregnancy and Prenatal Care in General

Columba migrated only seven months before I met her at Manhattan Hospital. She was twenty weeks into her fourth pregnancy. She left her elder three children in Ocuapa, Guerrero, in the care of her mother after asking her partner to help her migrate because of economic necessity: the remittances he was sending were not sufficient for their children's needs. At twenty-four years of age and one of the youngest of thirteen siblings, she was the only member of her natal family to migrate. She worked sewing in a textile factory. She told me that although she and her partner were *juntados*, as in a common-law union, she wished to marry him because she felt he might give her more financial support if they were married. As soon as the baby was born, she hoped to return to Mexico.

Columba told me her first three children were born at home, delivered by her mother. I asked her how her mother knew how to deliver babies, and she said that her grandmother had been a partera and her mother had herself given birth to thirteen children. When I asked whether her mother knew how to cut the umbilical cord and take care of everything, Columba said yes, of course, she did. Columba said that when she realized she was pregnant, a friend brought her to Manhattan Hospital. I asked Columba her opinion of the prenatal care she was receiving there. She told me that she felt it was too much: "Pues en México no nos están checando a cada rato y acá nos están checando siempre. . . . No pues a mí, no me gusta que me estén revisando a cada rato. Me molesto como no estoy acostumbrada" [Well, in Mexico, they aren't checking us all the time, and here they're always checking us. . . . And well, I don't like that they're always examining me. It bothers me because I am not used to it]. Columba indexes here a point of great variation in prenatal care: the "appropriate" number and frequency of prenatal visits in mainstream care varies dramatically around the world, with the United States ranking among the countries where the highest number of prenatal visits are recommended (Davis-Floyd et al. 2009; Ivry 2010; Strong 2000, 7). In fact, she said her solution was to avoid coming to all her appointments. She told me that she thought the pregnancy was normal and that she felt the same as with her earlier pregnancies. She did not see the need for constant examinations if her embodied experience was of a normal, uncomplicated pregnancy.

As discussed in Chapter 3, Mexican immigrant women in this study frequently described pregnancy as a normal, expected part of life that they are well equipped to successfully handle. Flora told me that she had no worries associated with her pregnancy; she simply wished to eat well, avoid frustration and anger, and take care of herself (see Ramírez Carillo 2001, 1). She thought that the care a pregnant woman requires is nothing special. Although Mexican women think that labor, delivery, and the postpartum period require certain specific interventions centered largely on enabling the body to rapidly recuperate and return to normal—avoiding *aire*, promoting the return of the uterus to its normal shape and size, restoring the abdomen and bone structure—they do not view pregnancy itself as inherently risky.

When I asked women what they thought they should do to ensure a healthy pregnancy, they frequently gave a short list of common recommendations. They reported consistency in the advice given them by their mothers, grandmothers, mothers-in-law, and also prenatal care providers. In addition to a common recommendation that they avoid *coraje*, becoming angry, and remain calm, *tranquila*, not to worry or become overly emotional, Mexican women had specific mandates that they repeated to me when asked what one needed to do to have a healthy pregnancy.[1] These are the "secrets" of a healthy pregnancy according to the women in this study:

- Eat well, but not too much.
- Walk a lot, but not too much.
- Rest, but not too much.
- Don't lift or carry heavy things.

This list is remarkable for its simplicity, as well as the activities that are not listed. For example, no one explicitly said that one should not smoke, drink, or do drugs. Alcohol, drugs, and cigarettes during pregnancy are the most prominent factors associated with low birth weight, after birth defects and chronic health problems in the mother (March of Dimes 2010). Virtually none of the women interviewed said that they consumed alcohol, drugs, or cigarettes during pregnancy (only two women said that they had one drink at a party during the course of their pregnancy, *para brindar*, in order to toast a special event) (see Sherraden and Barrera 1996). For some Mexican immigrant women, perhaps, there is no mandate to refrain from consuming alcohol, drugs, or cigarettes during pregnancy because to do so is unthinkable. Even though many of the women acknowledged enjoying a few drinks or cigarettes in conjunction with social occasions prior to or between pregnancies, this ceased during pregnancy.[2] Further, when I asked about difficulties they faced during pregnancy and their feelings about doing the things they thought they needed to do to care for their pregnancies, none mentioned abstention from these substances as a hardship. Judging from mainstream media debates in the United States about alcohol and pregnancy, whether "a half a glass of wine" or an "occasional beer" is safe, refraining from drinking alcohol during pregnancy is a guideline that is sometimes difficult for women in the United States to follow (see Hoffman 2005; Urban Baby 2010). For Mexican women, however, it seems understood, a given, that a pregnant woman will not consume such substances.

Walking was mentioned by many women in the study as an important part of pregnancy care. Virtually all the women said *caminar mucho*, walking a lot, is an important way to care for oneself during pregnancy. Although no one mentioned engaging in formal exercise regimens or more rigorous forms of exercise such as biking, swimming, or running, and they did not say that these were activities they thought they should do or refrain from doing during pregnancy, walking was almost universally discussed as an important healthful activity. Walking during pregnancy was described as a means to get the baby into a proper head-down position for delivery, to prevent excessive weight gain, to maintain strength needed for delivery, and to keep the baby from being *flojo*, lazy.

Walking during labor was said to speed dilation of the cervix and aid delivery. Some women even said they walked to the hospital during labor. As mentioned in Chapter 4, Nancy walked two miles to the hospital from her home during early labor with her husband and toddler. Lila, a bañera, said that she knew to walk during labor because her mother told her and her sisters to. Here she describes the dialogue between her mother and herself during labor:

> Porque mi mamá nos decía que cuando tuviéramos los dolores que no nos acostáramos, "¡Caminen, caminen, caminen!" Y es cierto es bien bueno eso. Llegábamos y caminábamos. "Acuéstate si quieres," me dijo. "No, yo quiero caminar," y caminaba. Y ya cuando tenía los dolores, "Ya ahora sí, me voy a aliviar."[3] "¿Y cómo sabes?" "Ya me voy a aliviar."

> [Because my mother told us, when we had labor pains, that we should not lie down: "Walk, walk, walk!" And it's true, that's really good. We got there and we walked. "Lie down if you want," she said. "No, I want to walk." And I walked. And when the pains came, I said, "Now, yes, the baby is coming." "And how do you know?" "The baby is coming."]

Perhaps her mother felt sympathy for her daughter's pain when she told her to "lie down if you want." But, with the walking, the baby descended so quickly into the birth canal that her mother questioned her, "How do you know [you're ready to give birth]?" She related that she just knew.

Women like Luisa, in Chapter 3, who had their babies in Mexico, described life in the countryside as more healthful in part because walking was a routine means of transportation; it kept women fit and strong for pregnancy, labor, delivery, and postpartum recovery. Although walking was also widely acknowledged as feasible and a routine part of life in New York City, Luisa, among others, said that one must make a greater effort to walk than in Mexico, that it is easier to be lazy.

Rest is related to exercise. Several women mentioned in interviews that if one does not walk enough or is otherwise too *floja*, her baby can also be lazy when born. The adjective *flojo* was used to describe babies who had poor sucking reflexes, who seemed "too sleepy" to nurse, or who were otherwise viewed as frail or weak. It was also thought that laziness could extend to adolescence and adulthood, that a woman who was lazy during pregnancy could have a lazy baby who would become a lazy adult, unwilling to do the work that life requires.

Many women described feeling lazy during pregnancy, especially in the first trimester, but they said they sought to conquer these sensations through activity and walking. Elba told me that if a pregnant woman "se lo pasa durmiendo el día, es más doloroso el parto, porque se les pega el bebé" [spends all her time sleeping, labor is more painful because the baby gets stuck to her]. To give in to feelings of sleepiness or tiredness was described as a failure to care for oneself and one's fetus. Even though many women ceased working early in pregnancy to care for their pregnancies, get rest, and avoid heavy labor, they described being as worried about the dangers of excess rest as they were about getting too little.

Refraining from carrying heavy loads and heavy exertion was frequently mentioned by women in the study. (Masley describes similar views among Mexican immigrant women in Ohio, 2008, 110.) It was widely thought that carrying heavy loads could result in a miscarriage or other damage to the fetus. This advice was often corroborated by providers in prenatal clinics. There seemed to be little controversy about the wisdom of this advice, although many women struggled to follow it given the demands of their daily lives. One woman said that she believed a miscarriage she experienced the year after her first child was born was due to lifting heavy things. Floridia told me that her cesarean scar opened following the birth of her first child because she had to get back to doing household work too quickly. In spite of this mandate, many women expressed concern that they had no choice but to do hard work and lift heavy objects, a fact that caused them distress. Many participants said they live in walk-up apartments, as many as six flights up. One woman said that she avoided carrying heavy objects by asking someone from the supermarket to carry her groceries up the four flights of stairs to the door of her apartment. Once she was there, her four-year-old son helped her by dragging the bags across the floor to the kitchen. María Pacheco, who lives in a fifth-floor walk-up, told me she had no choice but to carry her baby's stroller up the stairs, as her building was not secure enough for her to leave the stroller in the lobby. Other women described having to carry strollers with sleeping children up and down subway stairs or to their apartments. Others said that during their pregnancies, their partners carried laundry to the laundromat, carried groceries, and took their older children to school or the park so they could rest. But Emilia said, "Si no hago los quehaceres, ¿quién los hará?" [If I don't do the chores, who will do them?].

In Mexico, often more members of the family were able to share labor burdens and relieve a pregnant woman of rigorous tasks. One woman told me that her mother and mother-in-law argued about who got to take care of her after the birth of her first child. In Queens, however, she said, "No va a haber quien me ayude. Le traté de contar a mi prima, pero no acepta que es como una enfermedad que hay que cuidar" [There is no one who will help me. I tried to convince my cousin, but she doesn't accept that it is like an illness that one should care for]. However, some women said that in Mexico such burdens were worse, given demands from mothers-in-law to do domestic chores and given the routine labor required by a rural or semi-rural life with animals, homes, gardens, and children to tend.

Not only hard physical labor but all work is considered risky by some women. Even though working while pregnant is widely viewed by Mexican families as dangerous for the fetus, only one woman I spoke with was told by her medical provider to discontinue working outside the home during pregnancy. She had experienced break-through bleeding toward the end of her first trimester and was told that if she did not stop working and stay on partial bed rest, her pregnancy was at risk. In spite of their medical providers' silence about working during pregnancy, many women said that their partners and families encouraged and in some cases demanded they stop working. Pregnant women and their families routinely ignore that providers either do not have an opinion about working during pregnancy or encourage women to keep working until late in their pregnancy. Further, a man who insists his pregnant partner stop working is generally viewed as benevolent, as someone who takes proper care of his partner.[4] Women who insist on working generally do not do so within a frame of emancipation from machista demands but rather amid disclaimers about how their actions might be selfish and put their fetus at risk but are necessary for their own sanity and economic security.

María Pacheco had hoped to continue working during pregnancy, but her partner, Raúl, thought she should not. In her third month of pregnancy, she experienced bleeding while busing tables at the same soul-food restaurant where her husband worked. She went to the clinic and was told it was a normal complication. Shortly thereafter, while making collard greens, she felt faint, and the restaurant's owner told her to go home and rest. Raúl insisted she remain home for the rest of the pregnancy and asked his employer to double his shifts to compensate for the loss of household income. María was unhappy at home and often walked around the neighborhood for hours to avoid being cooped up in the apartment, but she was nevertheless grateful for her partner's concern.

Laura had a job folding tablecloths, which she described as light work, but when she experienced bleeding, her family insisted she quit. Mirna's partner insisted she quit her job sewing in a factory when she became pregnant, but only two weeks went by before she became desperate and begged to get her job back, unbeknownst to her partner. María and Laura described their partner's concerns in ways that indexed notions of modern, companionate marriage (Hirsch 2003).

Even though common biomedical discourses on risk are not commonly subscribed to by Mexican immigrant women, the grave risk posed by heavy lifting or excessive work during pregnancy was an exception to the idea that having a healthy pregnancy requires nothing in particular. Even though women in Mexico say that one can be excused from hard labor during pregnancy, they also argue that life in general there is characterized by hard work. Those women who are exempt from hoeing rows of corn or handling livestock still must wash clothes and hang them to dry, must scrub floors daily because of the penetration of dust in a rural environment, and must prepare food from scratch. In New York City, the ability to discontinue working during pregnancy becomes a form of status to some immigrants. In addition, some women said that if they were tired, they could get away with not sweeping the floor of their apartment, could do their laundry in coin-operated machines, and, occasionally, could ask their partner to pick up a roast chicken or Chinese food on the way home.

Although these characterizations are overly generalized—take-out food is available in all but the smallest villages in Mexico, and living in New York in a walk-up apartment with no laundry in the building requires quite a lot of heavy lifting—many women said that in New York they were able to do what they thought they needed to do to protect their pregnancies. Mexican immigrant families have some of the lowest average per capita incomes in New York City, but many women described themselves as having the resources they needed and being able to stop work without experiencing undue financial hardship.

Although additional research with their partners would be fruitful, it appears from women's comments that a man's ability to insist his partner stay home during her pregnancy is a luxury made possible by migration. Further, it is a luxury with greater value than other potential uses of resources. Although two women in the study said they lived alone with their partner—*solos*, or without apartment mates—the vast majority lived with their partners in apartments they shared with other families. The two women who rented apartments on their own with their partners also did not work during pregnancy. These trends and women's comments in interviews indicated it was considered more important for couples to use their resources to enable an expectant mother to stay home than to have privacy or additional space by renting an apartment for themselves. Although the sample in this study was small, it is notable that no one in the sample decided to continue working in order to rent an apartment alone.

Indeed, apartment shares were often credited with giving women the ability to stay home: because families shared domestic labor, childcare, and expenses, a pregnant woman could leave the workforce and care for the children of other women in the household who worked. When I asked women what they did not like about their living situation, the most frequent answers were conflicts over expenses and taste in foods. Privacy and space were only infrequently mentioned as issues, even though the women also often said that aspects of life they preferred in Mexico included having more living space. Further, although residence with extended family is common in Mexico, doing so does not always entail sharing precisely the same roof. María Pacheco's mother lives on the same property with her son, daughter-in-law, and their children, but her son built his own house on the land when he got married. A common phrase repeated to me was "la persona que se casa, casa quiere" [the person who marries wishes for his/her own home] (see Hirsch 2003; Pauli 2008).[5] Many families interviewed in this and a previous study (Gálvez 2009) describe their main objective for migration as the saving of funds to build their own house, frequently on family-owned land (see Gutmann 1996; Hellman 2008). Thus, living with extended family is not in itself valued as a long-term residential pattern by Mexican immigrants. It seems, then, that apartment sharing and its accompanying "crowding," which is cast as a social problem by some, is in fact a favored strategy in New York;[6] it enables families to obtain what they view as a necessary luxury: the ability for a woman who is pregnant to leave the workforce. (It also enables families to avoid hiring outsiders to care for their children, a fate many Mexican families seemed willing to do almost anything to avoid.)

Ideas about a Healthy Diet

Food played a tremendously important role in discussions of pregnancy self-care among Mexican immigrant women even though they said that one should simply eat what is "normal." Brenda described healthy eating this way:

> A nosotros nos gusta lo natural. En mi caso, mis hijos pesaron nueve libras. . . . Yo siento que todas las mexicanas comemos lo normal lo que es de siempre. Nosotros comemos comidas como nopales. En mi caso, a veces me hago un licuado de avena. A muchas mexicanas no les gusta la leche pero si comen lo que son tortillas, sopas, frijoles, carnes. O sea yo siento que ellas no son de tener una dieta, o sea, nosotros comemos lo normal.

> [We like everything that is natural. In my case, my sons weighed nine pounds. . . . I feel that we Mexican women eat what is normal, what we always eat. We eat foods like cactus paddles, and, in my case, I sometimes make myself an oatmeal shake. Many Mexican women don't like milk, but what they eat are tortillas, soups, beans, meats. I feel that most women are not going to have a diet; what I mean is we eat what is normal.]

Many women said they were told by family members not to eat pork during pregnancy and postpartum. Many were also told to eat a lot of fruit and vegetables and to avoid too much fried food. The following are the foods for which women told me they experienced cravings that they eagerly indulged: fruit (often with lime and chile), oatmeal, and licuados. The following are foods they told me they sought to avoid: pork, spicy foods, and fried foods. The most common foods women told me they consumed during pregnancy are *licuados de fruta o leche* (fruit or milk smoothies), yogurt, fruit, oatmeal, beans, eggs, milk, chicken broth or soup, stews, tortillas, and atole (a drink made of corn starch). Janette told me that she started to eat "normally" during pregnancy, that before becoming pregnant she had not cared for herself, eating only one meal a day. When she became pregnant, she said she had to think about her baby and could no longer be selfish.

Living in New York, many women overcame the food insecurity with which they were raised. Although many told me that at their family's table "nunca había suficiente" [there was never enough], after migrating, even though they were not rich, they could provide the basics for their families. Many women said, in New York, no one goes hungry. Even though the per capita income of Mexicans in New York City is among the lowest, by pooling resources in multifamily residential units and by taking advantage of public benefits like WIC, women said that they and their partners could provide enough for everyone to eat. Some remarked with wonder that in the United States, if one wants, one can eat meat every day. Many women said that they ate differently in New York than they did in their hometowns. Meat and poultry were generally viewed as more affordable, but fruits and vegetables were thought to be expensive and of poor quality: "Les falta sabor, ni huelen" [They have no flavor; they don't even have a smell]. Although resources to provide the basic necessities for a healthy pregnancy might be viewed as more plentiful in New York City than in Mexico, there are also factors that inhibit families' abilities to enjoy them; fast-paced lifestyles, demanding work schedules, and sharing kitchens with unrelated housemates were named by women as some of the factors constraining their ability to eat as they thought they should.

During pregnancy, weight gain is one of the most consistently deployed measures of satisfactory progress. Many women mentioned providing urine samples and being weighed as the most tedious parts of their regular prenatal visits. Pregnancy weight gain is overwhelmingly used as a measure in many Western prenatal contexts, whether with midwives or obstetricians, although it is not universal: Tsipy Ivry notes that in Israel many obstetricians dismiss weight measurement as a valid instrument for judging the progress of a pregnancy and do not engage in at all (2010, 70–71).

Because of the emphasis on weight gain and the high rates of gestational diabetes among Mexicans in the United States, excessive weight gain is a preoccupation for Mexican immigrant women during pregnancy. Rates of gestational diabetes among Mexicans in New York City rose from 2.5 percent in 1990 to 4.9 percent in 2001, a 96 percent increase. The citywide average for those years was 2.6 percent and 3.8 percent, respectively (Thorpe et al. 2005, 1537). Some of the increase may be attributable to statistical undersampling; in the 1990 sample only 2,916 women born in Mexico gave birth in New York City, whereas in the 2001 sample 6,780 women born in Mexico did. Nonetheless, Mexican women were described to me by providers as being especially prone to having gestational diabetes. In fact, rates of gestational diabetes for Mexicans (4.9 percent) are higher, according to Lorna Thorpe and her colleagues (2005), than rates for non-Hispanic whites (2.4), non-Hispanic blacks (3.1), and other Latinos (3.6–3.9), but lower than rates for Asians overall (7.4), South and Central Asians (11.1), and non-Hispanic Caribbeans (5.2).

Although having delivered a previous infant with macrosomia (excessive birth weight, over nine pounds) is a risk factor for gestational diabetes, and gestational diabetes can cause macrosomia, both lower and higher than average birth weights may lack pathology (Virginia Raugh, personal communication, 2010). When I described the birth-weight paradox to participants in this study, some women made comments along the lines of "Oh, es verdad, nosotras las Mexicanas tenemos bebés muy gorditos, muy sanos" [Oh, it's true, we Mexicans have chubby babies, healthy babies]. Chubbiness is viewed in this cultural context as a sign of health: a fat baby is strong and healthy, while a thin baby is viewed as *debilucho*, frail. It is in the public health care context that many women are told that having a heavy baby can be pathological or that having previously delivered a large baby is cause for increased vigilance from providers, repeat glucose tests, and sometimes assignment to high-risk prenatal tracks. As a result, weight and cultural assessments of it have come to occupy an important role in Latina women's negotiation of public services (Marisa Macari, personal communication, 2010; Emily Yates-Doerr, personal communication, 2007).

Further, many women told me that although, while growing up, they were concerned with getting enough to eat, they feared their children ate too much and ate the wrong kinds of foods. Concerns about obesity were prominent. Mothers told me they attributed high rates of obesity among Mexican children in the United States to consumption of comida chatarra, such as McDonald's, or eating pizza, French fries, and deep-fried chicken instead of homemade Mexican food; not eating as a family; rushed and consuming work schedules; demands on children like after-school programs; and a lack of exercise. Lack of exercise was attributed to parents' demanding work schedules and children being *encerrados*, closed up, in New York apartments and schools (Hellman 2008); harsh winters; and fears that if children spent too much time in the street, they would be exposed to gang recruitment, violence, drug abuse, and other urban hazards.

Although it was not part of my interview schedule, many Mexican patients brought up with me their regular visits to the WIC office at Manhattan Hospital. At these visits, women had to demonstrate continued eligibility for WIC benefits, a procedure requiring, among other things, that their children be weighed. Presumably a program designed to supplement nutrition would be focused primarily on ensuring that the benefits provided were being reflected in adequate nutritional intake by children. Many women told me, however, that far from being worried that their children were not showing sufficient growth, they experienced anxiety that their children would be found "obese." This anxiety arose not only because of concerns that their children's health could be compromised by obesity but also because such a finding would result in more frequent "weigh-ins" and scrutiny of their family.

In spite of efforts by federal administrators "to accommodate the cultural food preferences of WIC participants" (U.S. Department of Agriculture 2010), many women told me that they modified their eating habits to incorporate the foods they were eligible to receive within WIC, including what many viewed as excessive quantities of dried cereal, milk, peanut butter, and cheese, and a lack of other kinds of food they desired. One woman told me that the WIC counselor advised her that she should give her son only nonfat milk because he was gaining excessive weight. Further, because WIC is available only to children under the age of five, and food stamps are available only to U.S. citizens who meet income-eligibility requirements, many families with mixed status (typically undocumented parents and sometimes older children and U.S.-born younger children) creatively deploy food benefits to address the nutritional needs of WIC-eligible and ineligible family members. Others described using the WIC allotment of some household members to bargain for resources from others. For example, a mother who wished to stay at home with her infant, in addition to household labor might offer her housemates a share of the child's allotment of milk and dry cereal in exchange for being able to share in the groceries that employed housemates purchased. One mother told me, "Entre todos compartemos la leche, el queso y todo eso que viene con el WIC, pero ellos compran las otras cosas, y yo cocino" [We share the milk and cheese and everything I get with WIC among all of us, but they buy the rest and I cook]. Further, although many women told me they were not accustomed to eating so many "corn flakes," as some women called all dry cereals, they allowed their children to eat them as snacks but dedicated significant portions of their household income to buying larger quantities of fresh fruits and vegetables (which they described as very expensive) than allotted by WIC. One mother told me, "En México, a los niños les damos fruta, fruta, todo el día, pero aquí es un lujo" [In Mexico, we give kids fruit, fruit, all day long. But here it is a luxury].

Mexican women's attitudes about pregnancy weight gain and birth weight are under revision as they adapt what they consider signs of health and fortitude to conform to guidelines given them by prenatal care providers, pediatricians, and social workers. Janette, pregnant with her second child, described her experiences with her daughter, Stefany, who was fourteen at the time of our interview:

No fué muy gorda, pero fué muy sana. Entonces a mi realmente sí me molestaba mucho cuando venían y me decían que era muy delgada y todo mundo me fastidiaba: "Oye que está muy flaquita," que no sé, "¿qué no come?" y todo mundo me fastidiaba. Y me daba tristeza porque yo veía otros bebés, bebés gordos y hasta que un día hablé con una doctora y le dije: es que ella está muy flaquita. Me dice la doctora: "¿tu acabas de ver ese bebé gordito que salió ahora?" le dije que sí, y dice: "ese bebé tiene diabetes y está gordito y se ve bonito, pero no está bien, está en sobrepeso." Y luego tengo una amiga que tenía la niña de tres años y mi hija tenía siete, y tenía el mismo peso de mi hija, para tres años, y el sobrepeso. Tengo unas amigas, total que los niños tienen en la casa un montón de galletas, churritos—este—chocolates, y siempre están así como con mucho azúcar en su cuerpo, y siempre están empachados, siempre están devolviendo, y solo están encerrados en la casa, viendo la tele y muy hiperactivos, que desbaratan, todo lo contrario de lo que yo viví con mi hija, que nunca la he obligado a comer más de lo que ella puede comer y pues lo que le guste también, o sea no. . . . Mi papá lo que hacía era de "¡Coman!" y nos pegaba y de gritos y nos asustaba más y no comíamos, entonces nos volvíamos, como él decía, melindrosas, y con Stefany nunca he hecho eso y come de todo.

[She wasn't very chubby, but she was very healthy. So it really bothered me when people used to tell me that she was too thin: "Hey, she's too skinny," and, I don't know, "Doesn't she eat anything?" and everyone bothered me. And it made me sad because I saw other babies, babies that were chubby. Until one day, I spoke with a doctor. I told her, "My daughter is too skinny." She said to me: "Did you see that fat baby that just left here?" I told her I had, and she said, "Well, that baby has diabetes; he's chubby and he looks cute, but he's not well. He's overweight." And then I had friends, and their daughter was three years old and mine was seven, and she had the same weight as my daughter, meaning for three years of age, she was overweight. I have friends and they live in houses full of cookies, *churritos*, um, chocolates. And the kids are always going around with so much sugar in their bloodstream; they're always constipated and throwing up and always closed up in the house, watching TV and hyperactive; they're rowdy. And that is the opposite of what I experienced with my daughter. I never obliged her to eat more than she wanted to and made sure she ate what she liked, too. . . . My dad used to be one of those who would command, "Eat!" and he would hit us, shout at us, and scare us, so we didn't even want to eat. And my sisters and I became finicky, as he called it. With Stefany, I've never done that, and she eats everything.]

Here Janette describes her approach to food with her daughter as one of bucking the norms among her peers. At the same time, the conditions that she describes as contributing to children's weight gain are typical of migrant life in New York City (readily available processed foods, spending more time indoors than outside), not most of the places in Mexico from which migrants hail. Living in New York City, Janette has the option to both reject the aesthetic norms she attributes to other Mexicans that associate infant health and chubbiness, as well as the authoritarian parenting style that she describes scaring away her own appetite as a child. Thus, her contrarian stance toward the eating habits of other Mexican immigrant families affords her space to articulate an identity that is both modern and individualistic. Her migration has liberated her from the repressive parenting she associates with her upbringing, as, Matthew Gutmann notes, is common for people who are "remembering less-than-contented childhoods" (1996, 63). She makes the pediatrician who lets Janette into the secret that chubby babies may not be healthy an ally in her conceptual revisions. As such, Mexico and Mexican eating habits are cast as pathological and backward by Janette herself, even while the eating habits of the friends she describes are as much a product of migration as her own shifts in thinking are.

Views on Chemical Pain Relief, Medication, and Childbirth Interventions

Brenda told me her greatest worry in her first pregnancy was that she had perhaps inadvertently brought harm to her fetus by consuming cold medication when she thought she had the flu. When the medicine did not relieve her symptoms, she said that a member of her family told her, "You don't have the flu; you're pregnant."[7] She said she counted back the days to her last menstrual period and realized that it could be true. When she realized she had taken the cold medication at a month of gestation, she immediately made an appointment with the prenatal clinic at Coney Island Hospital.

Brenda and her husband told me about the home remedies they usually use to treat common illnesses. They said that if someone has a cold, they should be given a mixture of honey, grated radish, onion, and garlic, which works "like an antibiotic" to relieve a cough. They said they regularly gave their elder son tea made of cinnamon and onion for flu symptoms, as well, although they said cinnamon tea during pregnancy can be dangerous. For diarrhea, she recommended a tea made of corn silk. She referred to these practices as having a provincial origin: "Son tradiciones Mexicanas de provincia." Even though she and her husband were knowledgeable about and avid users of various home remedies, they dismissed others, such as avoiding lemon during pregnancy as *creencias* and *supersticiones*, beliefs and superstitions.

Although avoiding medication during pregnancy was not mentioned as often as the other mandates for having a healthy pregnancy, it was a common theme in interviews (see Root and Browner 2001, 210). Brenda told me that greater exposure to chemicals in the food and air in the United States made it more difficult for families to avoid using medications. She told me she had never heard of anyone suffering from allergies or asthma in Mexico, but in the United States she sensed it was a common problem. Claudia, from Castillotla, Puebla, received a great deal of advice from her mother and mother-in-law while pregnant. Her mother-in-law commanded her son to take good care of Claudia. Her own mother told her to drink hot water with lemon to boost her immunity and to use cool washcloths on her forehead if she had headaches. When she came down with a cold while pregnant and living in Brooklyn, she missed the herbal drops her mother bought for her from a naturopath.

In spite of what she described as a commitment to "todo lo natural" [everything natural], Claudia felt that a hospital birth was superior to a midwife-attended homebirth. Claudia and her siblings were born in a clinic, and she felt that having a baby in a hospital or clinic was the only safe and hygienic place to deliver. When I asked her why a clinic or hospital is better than having a child at home, she told me, "Pues están más preparados y tienen más experiencia, y está más desarrollado. Y estaba convencida de que iba a salir todo bien" [Well, they are more prepared and more experienced, and it's more developed. I was convinced that everything was going to turn out well].

The "natural-childbirth" movement in the United States is associated with a totalizing view of pregnancy and childbirth that rejects chemical and other interventions; advocates the use of women-centered birth attendants such as midwives, doulas, and the birthing woman's partner; and promotes breastfeeding (see *Mothering* magazine in general; Baer 2001, 2004; Belaskas 1992; Gaskin 2003; Maraesa 2003). This movement has provided the most prominent counterdiscourse to prevailing trends toward medicalization of childbirth and pregnancy in the United States over the last several decades. But, in spite of its history of activism, publications, and documentary films (Epstein 2008; Maraesa 2003), the majority of births in the United States do not comply with the characteristics associated with "natural childbirth." One widespread impact, though, may be the idea of "choice" in childbirth, in which women who subscribe to natural-childbirth notions as well as women who do not often discuss with their providers a "birth plan" in which they specify in advance their preferences regarding various interventions and pain-management techniques. This consumer-driven approach to childbirth, which extends, too, to the ways that women choose a prenatal care provider, is widely advocated in mainstream pregnancy-oriented periodicals as well as in advice books. Nonetheless, choice, or the illusion of it, is not equitably distributed and is rather more available to women with greater socioeconomic resources. Further, even though choice has emerged as a coveted value in health care, the reality is that birth in the United States has become increasingly characterized by medical interventions. In 2006, labor was induced in 22.5 percent of births, double the rate of 1990, and cesarean delivery reached a record high of 31.1 percent (Martin et al. 2009), while use of epidural anesthesia occurs in a majority of all births in the United States (Lane 2009).

"Natural childbirth" was not a movement any Mexican immigrant woman in this study professed an interest in or allegiance to. Nonetheless, many women in the study were assertive about their desire for what they called a "normal" or "natural" birth.[8] Brenda told me, "A nosotros nos gusta lo natural" [We like that which is natural]. When women asked me about my own childbirth experiences, one of the first questions they asked was frequently, "¿Los tuviste normal?" [You had them normally?]. I learned that by "normal" they meant a vaginal delivery, as opposed to a cesarean section. When I asked women in interviews whether they planned to have epidural anesthesia during labor, what some women called *la raquidia*, the way they phrased their response was typically "no, prefiero tenerlo natural" [no, I prefer to have it naturally]. Jessy told me that she preferred not to have anesthesia on the grounds that *antes no les ponían,* it was not done in the past. Leticia said she preferred to use her strength and have her baby "normally." She had an epidural with her first delivery but declined it with her second: "Me dijeron que con el segundo no era necesario" [I was told I did not need it with the second]. But with the third her labor was induced, and she was again given epidural anesthesia. She also told me that her biggest fear as she approached her fourth delivery was of the pain. Even so, some women, including Claudia, told me that they would accept an epidural if the pain became too much for them to handle.

Valentina Napolitano found in her research that women living in the metropolitan area of Guadalajara were more likely than their rural-dwelling mothers and grandmothers to accept pain relief during labor (2002, 166). Rural women saw "a positive connection between female endurance and the experience of coping in labor. For them, opting for a painless delivery undermines the central rite of womanhood" (166). She refers to the difference in opinion between older and younger and rural and urban women as "an intragenerational dialogical field where there is a tension of modernity between a self-choosing subject versus a reification of suffering and motherhood as a claim for agency" (166).

This difference seemed present in my study as well, but it correlated with recentness of migration, while Napolitano's data showed differences between rural and urban orientations. For example, although some women who migrated at an early age, before having children in Mexico, described wishing to try labor without anesthesia, they were less likely to reject an epidural out of hand than were more recently arrived immigrants and those who had previously given birth in Mexico. Women who had had children in Mexico, especially women from rural areas, irrespective of duration in the United States, were the most likely to express confidence in their ability to deliver their babies without chemical pain relief. Among the women in this study for whom I have data regarding their use of pain relief during labor, slightly more than 50 percent had an epidural during their most recent delivery, significantly lower than the rate of 58.5 percent nationwide for Hispanic mothers and 68 percent for all mothers (Martin and Menacker 2007, 6). However, far more than 50 percent told me in interviews that they wished to avoid an epidural. Although rates of epidural administration tell us nothing about desires to avoid or consume chemical pain relief, Mexican women who wish to avoid it may have more success than women from other groups.[9]

A significant percentage of women in the study told me they were opposed to having a cesarean section except in an emergency. Floridia told me she delivered her first child with a cesarean section at Metropolitan Hospital in Manhattan. I asked her whether she expected to have a cesarean with her second delivery.

Floridia: Yo quiero natural.

Alyshia: ¿Y le han dicho que sí es posible?

Floridia: Hasta ahorita no saben. Sólo me han preguntado como quería que sea.

Alyshia: ¿Y como diría que eran diferentes los partos de su mamá con él de usted?

Floridia: Bueno todo fue normal y fue en casa. Solo con partera particular.

Alyshia: ¿Y tuvo alguna complicación?

Floridia: Que yo sepa no. . . .

Alyshia: ¿Entonces no tuvo dolores con ella?

Floridia: Sólo un poco.

Alyshia: ¿Y le dijeron que iba a tener cesárea?

Floridia: Sí.

Alyshia: ¿Se estaba abriendo?

Floridia: Sí, pero dijo que no podía abrir bien.

Alyshia: ¿Le dijeron alguna razón?

Floridia: No.

Alyshia: ¿Y aquí le pidieron que trajera su archivo médico de Metropolitan?

Floridia: No me lo han pedido.

[*Floridia*: I want it to be natural.

Alyshia: And have they told you that is possible?

Floridia: As of now, they don't know. They only asked me how I wanted it to be.

Alyshia: How would you say your mother's experiences giving birth were different than yours?

Floridia: Well, everything was normal and at home. Only, it was with a private midwife.

Alyshia: Did she have any complications?

Floridia: Not that I know of. . . .

Alyshia: So you didn't have labor pains with her [indicating daughter]?

Floridia: Only a little.

Alyshia: And they told you that you needed a cesarean?

Floridia: Yes.

Alyshia: And were you dilating?

Floridia: Yes, but they said I could not dilate well.

Alyshia: And did they give you any reason?

Floridia: No.

Alyshia: And here, did they ask you for your medical record from Metropolitan?

Floridia: No, they haven't asked for it.]

Brenda told me her doctor asked how she delivered her first two children, who weighed more than nine pounds, without a cesarean. Karen had her first child with a cesarean at Sunnyside Hospital in Queens. Then she returned to Mexico where she had her second child. Her third was born at Saint Vincent's Hospital in Manhattan, and I met her during prenatal care for her fourth at Manhattan Hospital. She told me that in Mexico she was told that all her births would need to be via cesarean section because of failure of the incision to heal well. Indeed, all three were delivered by that means. However, with her fourth she still wanted to attempt to have her baby "normally," what providers refer to as VBAC, vaginal birth after cesarean. She was told by the providers at Manhattan

Hospital that if she attempted a vaginal birth, it would be at her own risk; they would not be held responsible. She told me, "Yo sé que puedo tenerlo normal" [I know I can have it normally].[10]

Rosario also sought to avoid a cesarean with her second delivery. Her first child was born with a cesarean section in a private clinic in Toluca, Estado de México. She was told that she was not dilating and her baby was not descending into the birth canal. With her second pregnancy, nine years later, her medical providers at Manhattan told her that she would likely need a second cesarean if she could not provide them with additional information about the reasons for the first one. She experienced symptoms of miscarriage and preterm labor between the fourth and eighth months of her pregnancy and was being seen by an ob-gyn because her pregnancy was classified as high risk. She asked her mother to withdraw her medical record from the clinic where her daughter had been born and to send it to her in New York. Her mother made two trips to the clinic but was unsuccessful in obtaining the records and was finally told that they were in storage or destroyed because nine years had passed. Rosa also told me she wished to avoid a cesarean as well as epidural anesthesia. She said she did not want marks on her body, and she wished to feel her baby.

In all these instances, women insisted that a vaginal birth was the only normal means of childbirth and expressed their view that a cesarean, far from being the routine procedure it is increasingly becoming in the United States, is an intervention reserved only for extreme situations. Nonetheless, they are given indications by medical providers that having a large baby without a cesarean is remarkable, that having a prior cesarean implies the necessity of future cesarean deliveries, and that any lacuna of data in their medical record can be grounds for a cesarean. In this way, their assumptions about childbirth being normal and natural except in extreme circumstances are challenged by clues that cesarean section is increasingly a default procedure.

Further, in these interactions, Mexico, and specifically Mexican health care, is constructed by providers as a place shrouded in mystery. Although some patients, like Rosario, went to extreme efforts to extract their medical records from Mexican hospitals and clinics, assuming that such records were comparable to the medical records that were being generated in New York City hospitals, I never observed that such records were seriously taken into account during their care at Manhattan. On the contrary, I frequently observed or was told by patients about the ways their efforts to inform their providers about past medical history were interrupted or ignored. Rosario, who insisted she was confident in her abilities to have a VBAC delivery and articulate about the reasons for a cesarean section with her first delivery, was told that her explanations were insufficient and that only medical records in a doctor's hand would serve to corroborate her story. Other women, who may have lacked Rosario's level of education and ability to explain in a medical vocabulary their prior medical histories, were less able to transmit the information about their prior deliveries that doctors viewed as relevant and crucial.

I was asked to translate for one doctor, Dr. Rose, the attending ob-gyn in the high-risk wing of the prenatal clinic, a woman who had a reputation for being especially brash and harsh with patients as well as with her medical students (Bridges, 2011, 162). Although the patient was not part of my study, I agreed to assist the attending physician. The physician had begun to take a history of the woman without translation but emerged from the examining room exasperated and calling for help. When I sat down beside her, the woman began to tell me a harrowing history of six pregnancies, only one of which had resulted in a live birth. She had experienced a few miscarriages and one stillbirth. One of the miscarriages was of twins. Dr. Rose was attempting to jot down the woman's story. Not a trained translator, I attempted to understand the woman's story for myself in order to translate it in a way that was comprehensible. Dr. Rose was impatient, insisting that I simultaneously translate, but then reprimanding the patient for being "loopy" and not having her story "straight." With the patient in tears, Dr. Rose asked, looking at me, whether the miscarriage of twins was the second or third pregnancy the woman had experienced. Parity, the number of pregnancies, is one of the first items to appear on a woman's prenatal care chart. "Multiparous," having had more than one pregnancy, and "primiparous" or "primigravida," or a woman's first pregnancy, are among the few tidbits of information relevant enough to appear on the prominent white board containing data about the in-patients in the labor and delivery wing. These numbers are clearly important to medical providers, but for the woman in front of me an accounting of her reproductive history was reckoned differently. The woman said she had lost four babies, given birth to one, and was expecting her sixth. She told me she miscarried her first pregnancy, then lost her twins—babies two and three—then gave birth to her son, before having a stillbirth. She was now several weeks into her sixth pregnancy. Dr. Rose became agitated and raised her voice as she insisted I put this information into a format she could use: first gravida, or number of pregnancies, then the outcomes of each of the pregnancies.

The way that Dr. Rose counted the patient's pregnancies and their outcomes and the order in which she wanted this information were not the same as the patient's, for whom babies—lost and born—were the central part of the story and pregnancies were secondary. In these interactions, it was clear that for at least some providers extracting medical histories from patients was considered an aggravating and inconclusive task. In this way, patients were given the message that their recollections of their own medical histories were unreliable and irrelevant to the care they received. Further, the emotional content of their stories was often pushed aside to make room for medical content. Although this attitude toward emotional content became most evident in interactions and differences of opinion regarding the medical necessity of repeat cesarean deliveries, it was also visible in other instances, such as when a woman tearfully recounted injuries her baby had received in birth but was interrogated for information that would indicate whether they were due to complications that were likely to recur.

Extramedical Interventions

Conducting research in New York City, I did not encounter or hear of a Mexican practicing midwife but did find nonpracticing bañeras, practicing yerberas, and a particularly renowned huesero, who does sobadas as well as some of the work traditionally associated with brujos. In addition to the care they receive in the public prenatal system, some Mexican women also solicit care from specialists who bring knowledge with which they were familiar in their hometowns. Often, care specialists are in fact from the same hometowns as their clients and operate on the basis of their reputation prior to migration. Women recounted seeking care from these specialists during pregnancy and after delivery for generalized aches and pains, sciatica, discomfort, incontinence, indigestion, skin problems, uterine cramps, and bleeding. They generally described this care as supplemental to their prenatal care, although sometimes they said it offered assistance that they could not obtain in a public clinic or hospital.

I was sitting in the administrative area of an after-school program in the Bronx run by an immigrant-serving institution when a man came in to give a massage to María Zúñiga, a friend and colleague who directed the program. She told me he had quite a reputation in the South Bronx. I learned, while he gave my neck a quick diagnosis and massage, that he was the huesero who had treated some of the people I knew, including María Pacheco.

María Pacheco's first baby was in a breech position at twenty weeks of pregnancy, and she was told by the high-risk practitioners at a Manhattan public hospital that she would need a cesarean section. Distressed and determined to have a vaginal delivery, she sought the help of the huesero. Over several visits, he manually turned her fetus. She told me it was painful but successful. She did not inform her prenatal care providers that she had sought outside assistance to turn her baby and ultimately delivered vaginally. External version, or external cephalic version, is a technique commonly known by midwives but rarely learned by obstetrical students in the United States today. It was mentioned by women in interviews as one of many strategies used by midwives in Mexico to avoid delivery complications. The same huesero gave María Pacheco massages to ease sciatica and other pregnancy-related pains. Some months after giving birth, she again solicited the huesero's help in relieving severe back pain, which immobilized her.

Perceptions of Risk and Mexican Immigrant Women's Responses to Them

The increasingly elaborate calculation of risk is one of the great accomplishments of contemporary epidemiology. Rather than make assumptions about healthfulness, behavior, habits, and genetics based on specious racialized categories and overly simplified health indicators, or subjecting all patients to a one-size-fits-all, prohibitively expensive and highly interventionist model of care, risk calculations allow a degree of customization based on specific indicators that an individual is likely to experience a given complication, disease, or other problem. Nonetheless, this grouping and categorization of individuals, presumably done to improve treatment, allocation of resources, and disease prevention, necessarily elides individual variation, while any logic of categorization can be questionable. Further, even setting aside the systems for categorization of social groups, calculation of risk in itself is not so transparent or objective as it might seem. Mary Douglas articulated an influential anthropological critique of risk as culturally embedded and socially constructed (Douglas 1985, 1992; Douglas and Wildavsky 1982). And Rayna Rapp, in her work on prenatal diagnostic testing, found a tremendous amount of variability in the ways that prenatal patients interpreted the calculations of risk made for them—such as the mathematical probabilities that a child might be born with a disability indicated in prenatal testing (2000; see also Bridges, 2011, 198; Glick-Schiller 1992; Layne 1996, 648n56; Martin 1994; Rabinow 1992; Susser 1973).

Mexican immigrant women may harbor different attitudes about risk than their care providers in public prenatal clinics do. Paola Sesia, as noted in Chapter 3, found that risk was a largely unknown concept for the Oaxacan midwives with whom she conducted research (1996). Mexican immigrant women living in New York City and consuming public prenatal care do not have the luxury to ignore epidemiological formulations of risk, but they may operate under different assumptions than their providers. Dorothy Nelkin posits that risk is a "surrogate issue, a proxy for many other concerns": "the way people interpret risks and benefits may be influenced less by the details of scientific evidence than by social, political, and ethical concerns, and especially by questions of participation and control" (2003, viii).

Indeed, in spite of being bombarded with constant information regarding the ways that their pregnancies were or were not anticipated to be "risky" in the prenatal clinic—the tracking of care into distinct high- and low-risk protocols, the frequency and mandatory nature of interactions with health educators, nurses, nutritionists, and social workers—Mexican immigrant patients sub-scribed to their own notions about the relative riskiness or lack of risk in their pregnancies. The vast majority of women reported that their mothers and grand-mothers (and sometimes their sisters and themselves) delivered babies without complications in settings far more technologically "primitive."[11] Mexican women who have been told they might consider additional prenatal diagnostic testing to determine whether they have a greater than average probability of chromosomal irregularities, for example, are likely to refuse such tests on the grounds that "no one in my family has had a baby with problems" and that, if anything, receiving technologically advanced medical care means they are at less risk than their female relatives in Mexico. Although they described life in New York City as posing certain challenges to their efforts to care for their pregnancies in ways that were familiar, it also brought certain benefits, especially increased buying power. Results from this study indicate that recent migrants may have favorable pregnancy outcomes in part because they do what they learned to do to care for their pregnancies from their mothers and grand-mothers, advantage also of the additional resources afforded by their own and their partners' better-remunerated work in the United States (Guarnaccia et al. 2010, 12).

Rubi told me that she thought the childbirth practices common to her hometown, San Felipe Xochiltepec, were better than the typical practices in New York City, although she expressed this opinion with a caveat. She said that in Mexico there was no option of anesthesia. Although she framed this lack as a shortcoming, she also said that anesthesia was not particularly necessary there. Although one gave birth at home with only "una señora que atiende en las casas" [a woman who comes to the house], the midwife took charge from early in the pregnancy of properly situating, *acomodar*, the fetus to minimize pain during childbirth. Rubi felt that if one really had a complication in labor and delivery, New York was a safer place than Mexico given the greater access to medical intervention, but she implied that such intervention was not neces-sary in a normal pregnancy. She said that the number of appointments to which she was subjected in New York was excessive and bothersome, but she knew when women had problems, they were immediately scheduled for additional protocols of care (see Bridges, 2011, 27).

Elva, a young woman pregnant with her first child who had migrated at the age of five, told me her mother was a midwife with a great deal of experience delivering babies in Mexico. Her mother was a great source of support and information during her pregnancy. In addition to offering her advice about diet and exercise, Elva's mother had palpated her womb and reassured her about the fetus's growth. This view contradicted the information Elva received at a public hospital in Brooklyn. When she went for her first visit, she was asked whether she wanted to abort the fetus.[12] She was later told that an ultrasound had revealed irregularities in the fetus and was given genetic counseling, which included information about abortion as a possibility. She said she and her husband were furious and withdrew their records and transferred to Manhattan Hospital. She said she had always had faith that the baby was fine. Elva continued her primary prenatal care at Manhattan Hospital. Nonetheless, she was so nervous that something might go wrong, she and her husband also paid out of pocket for consultations at a private obstetrical practice near their home in Queens. She told me the private doctor gave her more frequent ultrasounds and spent more time with her than her providers at Manhattan Hospital. Far from assuming her pregnancy was pathology-free, Elva felt pregnancy was an extremely risky proposition, for which she needed, in essence, triplicate prenatal care.

Although this study was not constructed to access those who seek prenatal care entirely outside the biomedical establishment, it does reveal that biomedical and traditional approaches to pregnancy care coexist for many women. In some cases, women and their families actively sought out the care of specialists, requested the shipment of herbs from their hometowns, and constructed make-shift temazcales in their apartment bathtubs. Soliciting the care of a huesero and, in particular, not mentioning that care to biomedical providers are indications that some Mexican immigrant women retain views of traditional medicine as valuable and efficacious. It would be useful for additional research to be conducted on what is likely to be a very small number of Mexican women who obtain all their pregnancy care and deliver their babies outside hospital settings in New York. In other cases, women did not actively seek out alternative care but operated under assumptions regarding their pregnancies and their abilities to deliver their babies without pain medication, cesarean sections, and other interventions, assumptions that ran contrary to the technoscientific approach they received in the prenatal clinic or the labor and delivery department. Many of the immigrant mothers I interviewed described changing their practices or choosing not to reveal their behavior to their providers in response to their anticipated opinions and preferences. In these ways, a disjuncture is evident between providers' assumptions about and approaches to the care of pregnant and laboring women and Mexican women's views about their pregnancies and labors. These disjunctures produce friction that may contribute to the wearing down of care practices or, at least in theory, their strengthening as a mode of active resistance to the subjectifying aspects of public health care.

Edwin Van Teijlingen and his colleagues write that there has been a "long-term worldwide evolutionary trend towards the medicalization of both child-birth and midwifery," which has led to a state where every pregnancy is considered to be at risk unless proven normal, an attitude that justifies the use of medical technology and intervention (2004, 2; see also Kleinman 1995). Even though their hometowns and states have been a part of this trend, many Mexican immigrant women do not unquestioningly accept that their pregnancies are risky. Their deeply held confidence in their own ability to produce a healthy infant is confronted by protocols of care that assume risk in ways that lead to an alteration in their practices and attitudes. In the next chapter, I contextualize these findings within citizenship theory.

Chapter 6

Prenatal Care and the Reception of Immigrants

Reflections and Suggestions for Change

Increasingly, long-term settlement by undocumented immigrants is reluctant: an artifact of the increasing militarization of the border and the closure of access to visa categories that in the past made circulation to and from communities of origin and migrant destinations feasible. As Douglas Massey and Magaly Sánchez write, "We have militarized the Mexico-U.S. border to block unauthorized migration, but this effort has reduced the outflow of migrants more than lowered the inflow" (2010, 246; see also Dreby 2010). Today, although not all unauthorized immigrants who find themselves living, working, and starting families in the United States do so because this is the place they would like to make their lives in the long term, the expense, legal risk, and physical danger inherent in travel out of the United States and back again (without documents) makes long-term settlement an increasingly favored option.

Since 1990, migration to the United States has become an ever more common option for those seeking to *superarse*, or overcome the odds they face in their home communities in Oaxaca, Guerrero, Puebla, and other states in Mexico (Cortes 2003). Through migration, families venture their well-being, financial stability, and fortunes on a journey north that is imagined, at the very least, to offer access to better pay (Massey and Sánchez 2010). In addition to the financial opportunities migrants expect to enjoy, migration has increasingly come to constitute a rite of passage (Gálvez 2009; Hellman 2008), a means by which young adults strive to project into being imagined, modern selves, often following several discursively constituted tropes (Dreby 2010; Hirsch 2003; Islas 2010; Napolitano 2002). These tropes frequently array around concepts such as modernity, responsibility, familial obligation, resilience, and hard work. This imaginative work is at least as important as the often backbreaking and exploitative labor that immigrants do in the United States. It is the aspirational labor of immigrants that inclines them to adopt certain attitudes and postures toward life in the United States.

Neoliberal Citizenship

The context from which immigrants originate is critically important. The Mexican state has failed to achieve its postrevolutionary promises of equality, prosperity, and development (Gutmann 1996; Napolitano 2002). Instead, it has designated the displacement of millions of former rural peasants, or *campesinos*, from subsistence agriculture as acceptable collateral damage within larger projects of "modernization."[1] Further, it has defunded and dismantled social safety nets as an integral component of neoliberal economic restructuring. Since the 1994 peso devaluation and the inauguration of NAFTA (to put an arbitrary start date on processes that began earlier), state policy has decimated rural economies, promoted industrialization, and rolled back state-funded social benefits, both to please multinational creditors and to comply with increasingly technocratic, neoliberal political trends that only increased with successive electoral victories of the PAN in municipal and congressional elections and, notably, in the 2000 and (disputed) 2006 presidential elections (Hellman 1995, 2008; Holmes 2009; Napolitano 2002). These trends have implied a withdrawal of some of the structural foundations for public health care in Mexico, at the same time that the nation's ongoing efforts to address high rates of maternal and infant mortality, among other challenges, have emphasized a "cultural approach," placing responsibility in the hands of individuals whose self-care, vigilance, and education are seen as the solution to their own and the nation's health problems (Maldonado 2010b).

Mexican immigrant women in New York were born in and grew up with a state that for much of the twentieth century failed to deliver the equality and state-funded social benefits outlined by the 1917 Constitution and promised by the revolutionary regime. Although strides were made in bringing health care to the countryside, that care has been couched within neoliberal discourses of modernity and progress. At the same time that these efforts have delivered certain services and professional expertise to previously underserved rural areas, they have also displaced traditional healers, including parteras.

Those who have experienced these vicissitudes of care the most are, of course, those who are always disproportionately affected by any feature of inequality: the poor. Although those with means have neither depended on nor mourned the destabilization of federally subsidized public medical care, the *clases populares*, popular classes, have long been accustomed to looking out for themselves and not only since President Calderón suggested they do so on International Women's Health Day (President of the Republic of Mexico 2009).[2] This depiction corresponds to Gutmann's description of the attitudes of residents of a working-class neighborhood in Mexico City: "a widespread belief that formal government institutions and officials could not be trusted to provide them with the necessities in life, and a general feeling that self-reliance was both the cross and the honor they would bear in life" (2002, 2). However, for people in communities that historically did not produce high levels of emigration, looking out for themselves increasingly requires elaborate transnational strategies. Although the truly abject poor still have little choice in such a consumer-oriented landscape, they are also largely unable to access that most spectacular of social safety valves, migration to the United States (De Genova 2009; Dreby 2010; Massey and Sánchez 2010). Those in the middle, those who describe themselves as having come from humble backgrounds but who nevertheless were able to marshal the resources to migrate, arrive in the United States having long managed their own and their family members' health. This self-sufficiency is reflected even in the etiologies of pregnancy, in which women and their family members—more than medical providers, genetics, or environment—are seen to bear the responsibility of caring for and producing a healthy baby.

A move toward "self-care" as officially promoted health care policy in Mexico has parallels in the trends that have resulted in a rise in immigration. Within both spheres, working families must look after their own physical, social, and economic wellbeing (Sointu 2006). They assume the risks and burdens of a migration project they imagine will, if it goes well, bring their family members on both sides of the border the economic and social stability and perhaps, mobility, that virtually all immigrants I have interviewed say they lacked while growing up.

The fact that these aspirations are often projected onto the next generation is not incidental: on the contrary, the sacrifices families make in the present for the imagined wellbeing of their children (who may not yet have been born) are a crucial component of their aspirational labors. As María Islas (2010) argues, through practices of transnational dreaming, people think about the future in ways that produce subjectivity in the present. This subjectivity is characterized by optimism about the opportunities migration affords, even in the face of experiences of exploitation, discrimination, debt, and family separation. This is what I call an aspirational stance, a posture that inclines Mexican migrants to view some of the benefits they accrue in New York, such as subsidized health care, public education, jobs, and apartments where three or four families can reside, as opportunities that, properly seized, can advance the family's overall project.

Within contemporary neoliberal state formations, citizenship is premised on a model of self-reliance. This model is related to what Foucault calls "technologies of the self," within which workers are constructed along with subjectivities in processes that both transform and reinforce power structures (1988; see also Besserer and Oliver 2010, 8, citing Tatiana Lara). Building on Foucault, Aihwa Ong identifies two key technologies for the formation of the neoliberal subject: *technologies of subjectivity,* "an array of knowledge and expert systems to induce self-animation and self-government so that citizens can optimize choices, efficiency and competitiveness" including health regimes and "other techniques of self-engineering," and *technologies of subjection,* "political strategies that differently regulate populations for optimal productivity" (2006, 6). Ong draws on Foucault's notion of "governmentality" as well as biopower: "the body as a machine: its disciplining, the optimization of its capabilities and the extortion of its forces" (2006, 13). Both these technologies are at work when Mexican immigrant women seek prenatal care in New York City's public health care system. Having long "engineered" themselves to be self-reliant, self-sufficient, flexible, adaptable, hard-working, and mobile laborers and caregivers, they enter public health care sites well-equipped to work wonders, achieving impressive outcomes in spite of a swath of statistically indicated disadvantages, including socioeconomic limitations (see Martin 1994). In this way, what began as a series of exclusions and disenfranchisements is sometimes recast as an honorable means for families to fortify confidence in their own resourcefulness and capability. Accompanied by pervasive concepts such as the preferability of modernity and its attendant models of family and residential arrangements, such neoliberal models of citizenship can be compelling indeed.

However, part of the work of neoliberalism is not to give credit to those who most successfully accomplish the kinds of self-engineering that decades of economic restructuring and adjustment have prepared them for—migrant workers and their families—but rather to penalize them, to discipline them into still more limited spheres of citizenship, where rights are reduced to consumption and belonging is ever more narrowly and elusively defined. As such, health care consumption becomes one site for performing modern neoliberal subjectivities at the same time as it implies the subjectification of immigrants and their children as unwanted subjects. In his description of the 2006 marches for immigration reform across the United States, Leo Chavez observes a counterintuitive narrowing of the sphere of public participation at the same moment when more immigrants than ever came "out of the shadows" to make claims for rights: "When immigrants marched en masse they performed the role of citizen subjects, but citizens of a particular sensibility: the economically contributing, entrepreneurial, government services-avoiding neoliberal citizen-subject" (2008, 18). The contradictions inherent in such a simultaneous expansion and delimitation of the scope of citizenship are present in health care encounters as well. As they consume public prenatal care, immigrant mothers are being offered models of ways to be that constitute an exceedingly narrow sphere of citizenship, constrained by neoliberal economic trends and racialized subject-making (Coutin 2003; Dávila 2008; De Genova 2009).

Contradictions in Immigrant Experiences with State and Medical Institutions

Undocumented immigrants' lives are often characterized by themselves and by others as being lived "in the shadows" as they seek to avoid detection by the state and those who might report them to immigration authorities. However, this characterization is overly generalized; it ignores the gendered dimensions of immigrant invisibility and visibility. Immigrant mothers' day-to-day experiences of seeking out services and resources for their children in public hospitals, schools, libraries, and welfare offices present an utter contradiction to the image of undocumented immigrants living clandestinely (Gálvez 2009). Accessing the benefits of the state requires full disclosure of one's address, phone number, medical history, "social history," income, living arrangements, marital status, employment, and—directly or implicitly—immigration status, among other information. Anahí Viladrich writes that through consumption of public resources, the immigrant family goes from being represented by "invisible subjects to [being] visible mothers" (2009). Any act of consumption of public benefits requires full disclosure not only of the identity and residence of immigrant families but also of their life stories and troubles. Families become accustomed to the contradiction inherent in these procedures: that one arm of the state can, and must, know everything about one's life; while another, Immigration and Customs Enforcement (within the Department of Homeland Security), must know nothing.

Recipients of public benefits also become accustomed to the contradictory postures that are necessary for access: that is, they must simultaneously demonstrate both need and worthiness even though doing so, in many instances, runs contrary to their instincts to demonstrate they are capable of caring for their families themselves. When Mexican women are asked about the food they eat, their social networks, income, living situation, and expertise as mothers by those public employees charged with disbursing services to them, their first instinct is often to demonstrate their ability to resolver, in spite of humble means (Gálvez 2010). They are obliged to demonstrate need as a first access point to services that may aid them even though they simultaneously subjectify them. At the same time, they must perform their willingness and ability to appropriately care for their children in spite of economic constraints. If this capacity is questioned, they make themselves eligible for increased scrutiny and even intervention by ACS. Yet, if they too effectively demonstrate their abilities, they will be ineligible for the services that most of them feel they need: medical care and nutritional assistance. Thus families become ensnared in a tenuous cycle of performances of need and performances of capacity.

From their mothers, many immigrant women describe having learned to be strong, resilient, and resourceful. Their attitudes about pain medication during labor and childbirth are only one example of the many ways that women have been socialized to believe their bodies are already capable of successfully bearing children with little expert intervention or supervision. As eager as they are to overcome what many view as the demeaning circumstances of their mothers' childbirth experiences—en la casa, en el suelo, con una partera—by accessing what they view as a superior, more modern, and more humane health care system in New York City, they still see some aspects of the care they receive in that system as excessive and constraining. The hypervigilance of prenatal care providers—the number of prenatal visits, exams, tests, and diagnostics—was described by some women as bothersome. The mandates received by some to facilitate the measurement and surveillance of the progression of their labor by remaining prostate and consenting—frequently without being given an explanation or alternatives—to minor and major interventions during labor and childbirth destabilized their understandings of themselves as capable of having uneventful and "normal" deliveries. They were encouraged by hospital personnel to conform to culturally constructed expectations that Mexican women should be docile and stoic and have a high pain threshold at the same time that the circumstances in which they labored and gave birth left little room for their own culturally constructed ideas about pregnancy and childbirth, such as the necessity of walking during labor and delivering in an upright position. Just as achieving eligibility for benefits requires certain performances of need and docility, the technocratic model of birth requires subjectification and alienation from the embodied experience of pregnancy. As Bethany Hays has written, "Relinquishing one's personal power is a prerequisite for obtaining the gifts of modern medicine" (1996, 292; see also Martin 1992).

Although providers generally have positive attitudes about Mexican patients and are familiar with the birth-weight paradox, which is currently all the rage in some public health and epidemiological circles, these understandings rarely alter the course of women's care. If the paradox consists of better-than-expected results, women are still being incorporated into protocols that anticipate worse-than-average outcomes. Khiara Bridges calls this practice "pathologizing as an equalizing move" (2011, 26). Mexican women are viewed by providers as healthy and prone to take good care of themselves during pregnancy, but this view does not earn them a pass when it comes to protocols for care. Those protocols are based on calculations of risk that predict that Mexican immigrant women, with low rates of health-insurance coverage, low socioeconomic status, low rates of formal marriage, high rates of "teen" pregnancies, low levels of education, are likely to have pregnancy complications. These risk profiles do not differentiate between Mexican immigrants and women who were born in the United States; they do not always differentiate even between Mexicans and other Latin American–origin groups. Risk calculations do not take into account the protective features that research has shown enable Mexican immigrant women to defy the socioeconomic and structural odds and enjoy fewer pregnancy complications than do women in many other groups. This is not to say that risk and racial profiling of mothers of other groups is acceptable or legitimate, it is simply to point out the utter inadequacy and, at times, violence of a one-size-fits-all approach to prenatal care that spends more time grouping women and analyzing their risk factors than inquiring into their preexisting knowledge about pregnancy, care practices, habits, and health history. As a result, the wearing away, sloughing off, and outright rejection of those protective features by many immigrant women patients themselves is frequently neither noticed nor mourned.

The public prenatal care system in Manhattan Hospital, where I conducted participant observation, as well as in other hospitals where interviewees received prenatal care, is oriented around assumptions of need and risk. Congruent with Aizita Magaña and Noreen Clark's (1995) notion of the "assumption of minority dysfunction," Mexican immigrant patients not only are expected but are required to demonstrate need in order to qualify for the services they desire to access. Further, the processes by which individual patients and their families assert need in order to access services concurrently constructs their group—Mexican immigrants—as a collective that is, on the whole, needy. In turn, such a construction narrows the realm of interactions with health care professionals available to future ostensible members of the group, other Mexican immigrants. This construction of "groupness" constitutes racialization (which I discuss in detail below), and it happens in the context of ever-shrinking public resources for health care, education, and other services: "As minority groups are compelled to compete amongst themselves for decreasing amounts of money and political support, they also compete to present their communities as the most dysfunctional" (Magaña and Clark 1995, 100).

Subtractive Health Care: The Loss of Protective Features in Pregnancy and Childbirth

In her study of a public high school with a majority of Mexican and Mexican American students in Houston, Texas, Angela Valenzuela built on social-capital theory and subtractive-assimilation literature to develop her concept of subtractive schooling: "For the majority of Seguín High School's regular (non college-bound) track, schooling is a subtractive process. It divests these youth of important social and cultural resources, leaving them progressively vulnerable to academic failure" (1999, 3). Building on Robert Putnam's concept of social decapitalization (1993), she found that "the systematic undervaluing of people and things Mexican erodes relations among students, as well as between teachers and students. Cultural distance produces social distance which in turn reinforces cultural distance" (1999, 20). At Seguín High School, educators, many of whom described themselves as caring and committed, contributed to the reproduction of inequality.

In Manhattan Hospital, I observed well-meaning prenatal care providers reinforce dominant stereotypes and derogatory assumptions about Mexican patients, even while acknowledging and marveling at the birth-weight paradox. A prenatal encounter that allows no time or opportunity for women to share the practices and attitudes associated with pregnancy and childbirth that they bring with them from their rural communities can result in the loss of those practices and attitudes. Further, the "assumption of minority dysfunction," made not only by providers but by the entire web of public health care institutions from the moment a patient initiates enrollment in Medicaid (PCAP), reinforces the characterization of such patients as, at best, empty vessels that must be filled with instructions and mandates or, at worst, pathological and poor, unwilling and incapable of following any but the most basic and diluted medical advice. Unrecognized, out of place, and invisible, the practices and knowledge women bring with them are marginalized and eroded.

Although for some women, presumably, the eligibility screenings for PCAP and intrusions into their decisions about contraception, family size, home life, diet, economic resources, relationship with their partner, living situation, and more are merely bureaucratic hoops to be jumped through—with little impact on their notions of self or their practices—for others, the stakes are greater. The required childbirth-education classes and visits with social workers, nutritionists, and nurses offer a means of socialization into what is expected of these women—as patients, as mothers, as consumers of public services, and as citizens. Nurses and physicians' assistants who speak to the women in their own language are often the ones who deliver socializing messages: that they need to behave like Mexicans are expected to; that they should not complain or make trouble; that they should follow instructions; that they need to stand up to their husbands and have their tubes tied, use "la inyección" or "la T de cobre";[3] and that they will fail at all of this and be back again next year with another pregnancy.

Even though scholarly hypotheses about the birth-weight paradox center on the "cultural advantages" of Mexican immigrant women, culture has no place in the clinic. Moreover, in a technocratic, ostensibly neutral medical establishment, culture can be viewed as a liability: the elusive positivist goal of full predictability and manageability of risk factors and care protocols leaves little room for the subjective or the intersubjective. Because no site is fully technocratic and calculations of risk have yet to achieve full scientific verifiability, objectivity, and neutrality (and, cultural anthropologists would widely agree, never will), the slim space left for interpersonal interaction in the prenatal encounter is too often filled with subtractive processes rather than additive ones.

In this way, the ideas and practices about pregnancy and childbirth that have been associated with favorable birth outcomes among recent immigrant women from Mexico are rapidly stripped away. This stripping away is not done entirely to Mexican patients but also by them as they slough off the habits and self-care technologies that many associate with a lack of options and poverty. Even though their fundamental etiologies of pregnancy—the ideas they have about their abilities to conceive, carry, and deliver a healthy baby—seem to remain largely unshaken in the first generation, Mexican immigrant women quickly amend the practices with which they care for their fetuses and give birth to their babies to adapt to what they view as a modern and technologically superior approach to pregnancy care. Such adaptation can be seen in their embrace of hospital births. In spite of popular understandings in U.S. urban contexts of public hospitals as providing inferior care and services compared with private hospitals and of public insurance as affording less care than what one might access with private insurance, Mexican immigrant women are not always aware of these hierarchies. On the contrary, they compare New York

City's public health care system with what they remember from Mexico in the 1990s, when having a baby in a hospital or clinic was a privilege for the better-off and virtually everyone they knew delivered with a midwife because of a lack of options many described as preferable. In this way, the important distinction between births has to do with delivering at home or delivering in a hospital, not delivering in a public ("bad") or private ("good") hospital as women dwelling longer or born in New York City might view it. Valenzuela calls immigrants' "dual frame of reference" an "enabling quality that allows immigrant[s] to compare their present status and attainments to their typically less favorable situation 'back home'" (1999, 14; see also González 1986, 242–243). Mexican immigrant patients do not always realize that the health care they are being offered is viewed by many others, including providers, as basic, "shoestring," even inferior (Bridges 2011). Meanwhile, providers in Manhattan Hospital describe themselves as "working in the trenches" and "being on the front lines," as sacrificing higher-paying and higher-status private practices, often because of a professed commitment to equality and social justice in health care and in the spirit of serving the needy.

The adaptations in care that Mexican immigrant women make are related to findings in public health literature on the effects of racialization. As described by Arline Geronimus, the "weathering hypothesis" principally posits that some women's health "may begin to deteriorate in early adulthood as a physical consequence of cumulative socioeconomic disadvantage" (1992, 207). Geronimus's research was based on infant mortality rates for African American women, but the theory is productive for analyzing the changes in Mexican women's care practices during pregnancy and childbirth. This research and related studies (Conley, Strully, and Bennet 2003; Borrell 2005) offer potential insight into the biological pathways of social inequality: How is it that poverty and disadvantage get into the body and result in poor health outcomes? Luisa Borrell writes that even so seemingly benign an act as checking one box rather than another on a census form can have a clinical impact on health: "It is possible that categorizing Hispanics into U.S. Census racial categories channels them toward or away from opportunities and resources that may influence their life chances and, further, their health status. Thus, categorizing Hispanics within the racial categories Black or White could confer on them socially-patterned experiences and exposures similar to those of non-Hispanic Blacks, thus affecting their health negatively and leading to disease, disability and death" (2005, 380).

The process of categorization into racial categories, also known as racialization, can have a detrimental impact on health care. Although my research does not examine the racial identities or classifications of patients, it is clear that Mexican immigrant women in New York City's public health care system experience racialization: a process of socialization from immigrants into patients and then into racialized minorities. Bridges calls pregnancy, especially when viewed in the context of public health care, "a racially salient event" (2011, 19). The process of racialization may have detrimental impacts on the quality of care given by providers as well as on self-care, as immigrants come to think of the practices they have always engaged in as ill-adapted to their new environment. Although studies of the birth-weight paradox have traced the erosion of Mexican immigrants' cultural advantage over generations (Cobas et al. 1996; Guendelman and Abrams 1995; Scribner 1996; Scribner and Dwyer 1989; Wilson 2008) in ways that lend credence to the racialization hypothesis, they have overlooked the key life stage and posture this book examines: the period in which recent Mexican immigrants reconcile conflicting advice and care practices with their own aspirational stance as well as with larger societal ideas about immigrants.

Dalton Conley, Kate Strully, and Neil Bennet (2003) found that the seemingly biological fact of low birth weight can be caused by factors that are both biologically and socially inherited: "The social condition of poverty inherited across generations may also be an independent factor behind family patterns of low birth weight" (2003, 16). An infant with a low-birth-weight father is 975 percent likelier to be born with a low birth weight than an infant born to a non-low-birth-weight father; for infants born to mothers who were themselves born with low birth weight the chances are 555 percent higher than for those with a non-low-birth-weight mother (2003, 56); but Conley, Strully, and Bennet show—through rigorous data analysis that I am unable to adequately reproduce here—that this correlation is more likely caused by inheriting poor life chances than by any direct biological, genetic factor. In fact, they argue that it is possible that causality is the reverse of that which is assumed: rather than class causing health status, health may be determining socioeconomic status (2003, 77). Infants born to a parent who was himself or herself challenged by low birth weight is significantly more likely to start life with the same challenges; thus, according to Conley, Strully, and Bennet, disadvantages are perpetuated that are biological and also socioeconomic.

Prescriptions

The Mexican population in New York City is relatively recently arrived. Although interactions in public hospitals and other institutions do not exist in a vacuum, immune to general discourses about immigrants, pluralism, cultural diversity, and more, New York City is a place that generally prides itself on being pro-immigrant, and negative discourses about immigrants still have limited currency. Recognition of Mexican immigrants' contributions to the city is not unusual or terribly controversial. Presumably, if the ideas and practices with which Mexican women enter the public health care system can be reinforced and valorized by providers rather than marginalized and ignored, they can be added to the repertoire of care practices available at Manhattan Hospital. This should be done with and for not only Mexican patients but all patients. Although some ideas that women may have about pregnancy care are not corroborated by best practices in obstetrics and some may have a neutral impact, many others are solidly beneficial.

Rather than submit women to an excessive number of short, intrusive, and bothersome prenatal exams, prenatal care could be reoriented to refresh and reinforce existing healthful notions about pregnancy and fortify women's understandings of their own abilities to deliver a healthy baby. A fewer number of prenatal visits could be interspersed with collaborative workshops, attended by patients, midwives, physicians' assistants, medical residents, and physicians. Led by neutral facilitators, including leaders of community organizations, these workshops could focus on topics such as conception and fetal development, social support, nutrition, balancing the needs of older children during pregnancy, aches and pains in pregnancy, labor and delivery options and pain management, and postpartum care. In these workshops, organized into language groups or conducted with translators, patients could share their own ideas about pregnancy, develop ties to other women pregnant at the same time, and reinforce ideas and practices with which they enter the prenatal encounter.

Important research has examined health disparities by examining barriers to access typically experienced by poor, racialized minorities and immigrants; other research has argued for increased cultural competence among public health care professionals and cultural sensitivity in models of care (*Access Denied Blog* 2009; Eckersley 2006). Few of the women in this study described prohibitive barriers to access.[4] This is a finding at least in part skewed by the fact that my primary research site was a public prenatal clinic where women were by definition already inside the public health care system. Further, access varies widely state to state, and New York is routinely recognized as one of the most generous states in offering free or low-cost prenatal care to women regardless of immigration status. Yet, cultural sensitivity from providers was certainly lacking in many of the interactions women described. Jennifer Hirsch critiques the insertion of culture as an inadequate solution to health disparities in public health settings: "Culture, and its programmatic corollary cultural appropriateness, have been embraced because they are an easy pill for us to swallow in public health. They suggest that if we capture just the right cultur-ally appropriate perspective, [if] we could just tell people how to be healthy in the right words, they would listen and all would be well" (2003, 274). She argues that instead of "asking people to make themselves healthier, one by one by one," public health must take into consideration the political economy of health (2003, 274; see also Santiago-Irizarry 1996). Other scholars have argued that cultural competence is an important and valued corrective to clinical prac-tice, while also arguing that it needs to be more nuanced and sophisticated in its conceptual elaboration of the notion of "culture" (Guarnaccia and Rodríguez 1996, 420; Escobar and Vega 2006).

I would argue that a better approach to Mexican immigrant women's health care would start, first and foremost, by acknowledging in implicit and explicit ways that Mexican women are likely to already have the tools and knowledge needed to achieve a healthy pregnancy and birth. Although there is vast diver-sity, even among Mexican immigrants, in rural and urban origins, level of edu-cation, exposure to traditional birth practices, and more, women in this study demonstrated remarkable continuity in their basic, sound prescriptions and atti-tudes about pregnancy, childbirth, and postpartum care. This knowledge ought not to be ignored or marginalized in the prenatal encounter. Instead, prenatal care could take a rather more inquiry-based approach, which would be unlikely to increase costs or expenditures of time and might even offer savings in these areas. If a woman complains of nausea, she could be asked, "Do you know of any solutions to nausea during pregnancy?" If she suggests, as Marisol did in the opening vignette of this book, that nausea in her first pregnancy subsided when she ate fresh chicken soup, she could be told, "That sounds like a great idea!" Women's preferences surrounding chemical pain relief, positions for labor and birth, and more should be heeded, noted in their files, and discussed when they arrive to deliver their babies and throughout labor and birth rather than being trampled by biomedical protocols and doctor-led interventions.

The knowledge and inclinations with which immigrants enter the public health care system are eroded by processes of racialization, assumptions of minority dysfunction, and subtractive health care. Immigrant women leave behind the protective practices that have enabled them to enjoy better-than-expected pregnancy outcomes not because these practices are deemed haz-ardous by providers but because women themselves do not see them as well-suited to their lives in the United States. As women are socialized into the public health care system in New York City, they leave behind many of the habits and attitudes they are familiar with in their home communities. They view the intervention-filled model of prenatal care and delivery that predominates in the United States, and increasingly in Mexico too, as safer and more modern than care as they remember it in Mexico (see Sargent and Bascope 1996, 215). Freed from the obligation to care for themselves, they view the health care services they consume as benevolent and humane. The ways that women in their home communities cared for their pregnancies are rejected as a shameful legacy of poverty and disenfranchisement, a failure of the liberal state to provide for its members, and a result of neoliberal structural adjustments premised on *autovigilancia,* self-vigilance, and *autocuidado,* self-care. In this way, Manhattan Hospital becomes, for both patients and providers, a sanctuary from neoliberal conceptualizations of citizenship: a liberal haven in an increasingly neoliberal age. But even while the hospital offers progressive social goods, it does so within larger neoliberal logics that are external (globalization, transnationalism, and migration) and internal (cost-cutting, social hierarchies of immigrants and citizens, and the increasing brunt of responsibility for self-care).

The effects on the body of racialization are not clear, and much research remains to be done to definitively trace a relationship between forces like subtractive health care, segmented assimilation, racialization, weathering, and declining birth outcomes among women of Mexican origin. Nonetheless, the present study suggests that strategic efforts in public health care sites could have an immediate and favorable impact on the retention of protective cultural practices during pregnancy and childbirth. Although the authoritative knowledge of technocratic models of birth have been found in the anthropology of reproduction to disempower women, in this case the authority of prenatal care providers could be turned to empowerment and additive health care. Aspirational narratives among immigrants place a premium on health care models available in the United States that are perceived to be modern and technologically superior and often imply a denigration of the self-care practices to which families historically resorted in their hometowns. Medical care providers could utilize their esteemed position not to subtract from but to reinforce the healthful practices with which many Mexican immigrants enter the health care system.

Immigration status in itself has begun to be acknowledged as a key factor in analyses of perinatal advantage (McCarthy et al. 2005), a vast improvement over the methodology of previous studies, which did not disaggregate Mexican-born from U.S.-born women of Mexican descent. Nonetheless, declines in the Latina perinatal advantage over the course of individual women's reproductive lives have yet to be identified in research.[5] Although Mexican immigrant women who have been in the United States for decades still show lower rates of low birth weight and infant mortality than those in second and succeeding-generations, whose outcomes resemble those of other similarly situated socio-economic groups, it is likely that Mexican immigrant women with shorter duration in the United States retain a comparative advantage over women who migrated earlier. Although this study was not large enough in scale to reveal the perinatal outcomes of a statistically significant number of both recently migrated women and women who migrated previously, it does clearly reveal that women in this sample are rapidly leaving behind many of the practices that have been hypothesized to confer benefits to pregnancy outcomes. They are often pleased and then perturbed at the frequency of visits and the intru-siveness of health care providers who question their eating habits, parenting, self-care practices, and even basic conceptualizations of their own ability to grow a healthy fetus. Women who experienced what they describe as normal, uncomplicated home births in their hometowns in Mexico express surprise and dismay at the complicated twists and turns their labors and deliveries take in New York City hospitals, where Mexican women wind up more than half the time with epidural anesthesia and labor augmentation, and, in many cases, with cesarean sections.

The biological pathways of such social changes are far from clear, and women's health may not be declining between earlier and later pregnancies more than can be expected because of advanced maternal age. Differences in birth experiences may be the result of a more medicalized approach to labor and childbirth in which interventions are more frequent and routine. Nonetheless, while wincing from the pain of a cesarean incision or rubbing the bruises left on their baby's head by forceps, women wondered, and asked me, what went wrong. The results of these processes of change do not bode well.

As Mexican immigrant women's pregnancy outcomes begin to more closely resemble those of others who share their socioeconomic status, health-insurance coverage, and prenatal care consumption rates, statistics indicate that public efforts to continue to lower infant (and maternal) mortality rates and rates of low birth weight will be challenged by rises in these indicators among one of the few groups that enjoys relative protection from them. Although the weathering and racialization hypotheses and theories of segmented assimila-tion indicate that immigrant socialization for those who are members of racial minorities without high levels of social, educational, and economic capital can be a downward process (Massey and Sánchez 2010; Portes and Rumbaut 2001; Portes and Zhou 1993), this outcome is not inevitable. Identifying the factors associated with favorable pregnancy outcomes among Mexican immigrants should lead to a promotion of those factors and of efforts to prevent the denigration of the practices and attitudes associated with healthy pregnancies. Viewing their rural hometowns as anything but backward and the repository of youthful dreams can be difficult for immigrants who have made such massive sacrifices to come to the United States. Nonetheless, pride in their cultural background and the wisdom of their mothers and grandmothers can be promoted and, perhaps, preserved. At the very least, they can find a place in the prenatal care encounter, rather than being marginalized by and subtracted from interactions with providers.

Citizenship

Contemporary definitions of citizenship used in immigrant-receiving nations are arguably narrower and more juridical than at any other point since the American and French revolutions. Suzanne Oboler writes: "Increasingly, citizenship has been conceptualized primarily in juridical terms in relation to noncitizens and (im)migrants, even while the state is strengthening its prerogatives in narrowing both the practical scope of the rights and benefits granted under this particular entitlement and the beneficiaries, especially in relation to noncitizens" (2006, 5). As constitutional scholar Alexander Bickel (1975, 36) points out, citizenship is nowhere defined in the U.S. Constitution. Although undocumented immigrants are fully aware of their exclusion from the benefits and privileges of juridical citizenship, they aspire to fair treatment and dignity in the place where they have migrated to work and, often, to live in the long term.

Citizenship has historically been gendered both in explicitly exclusionary ways (exclusion from the vote) and implicitly within discursively constructed notions of the (male) citizen-subject. Nira Yuval-Davis and Pnina Werbner signal the "apparently intractable opposition posed by feminist critical theory between abstract universal egalitarianism (masculine), and particular discourses of needs and care (feminine)" (1999, 7; see also Pease Chock 1996). Some scholars have found theoretical exits from this dilemma: Joann Martin writes about the "importance of the mother-child bond as a model for reconceptualizing politics" (1990, 470); Jennifer Schirmer (1993) and Werbner (1999) write about "political motherhood." Further, empirical realities—a feminization of migration, for example (Hondagneu-Sotelo 2003)—challenge in real time old conceptualizations of agency, subjectivity, and citizenship. Nonetheless, historically, splits between public and private, between male and female, and between provision of goods and services and consumption of them have been enduring. In an explanation of the historical antecedents of discourses of citizenship in the United States, legal scholar Kunal Parker writes that in late-eighteenth-century Massachusetts, indigent persons could be expelled from towns when they made demands for relief (2001). Although "citizenship/subjecthood" was not a prerequisite to territorial rights, failure to properly document settled residence could lead to an exclusion from social benefits (2001). The receipt of welfare benefits has long been noted by scholars as a justification for loss of autonomy (Pease Chock 1996; Piven and Cloward 1971).

Similarly, today, consumption of benefits is argued by many to constitute a reason to bar immigrants from regularization of their status, including naturalization. This was the spirit behind the 1996 Illegal Immigration Reform and Immigrant Responsibility Act, which bars legal permanent residents from consumption of public benefits like food stamps, Medicare, and Medicaid for five years (Hoffman 2006, 240; Viladrich 2009). Although largely ineligible for any benefits except during pregnancy, undocumented immigrants are widely aware that consumption of public benefits, which they often refer to under the catch-all term *welfare,* can cause them trouble if they later seek to regularize their status. For this reason some choose not to enroll in programs like PCAP and WIC during pregnancy and for their young children, despite need and eligibility and even though consumption of such benefits is generally excluded as a reason for barring an adjustment of status. The use of public services by immigrant families has become the most volatile issue in immigration debates in the United States.

Phyllis Pease Chock (1996) traced the discourse surrounding immigrant women's fertility and consumption of public services in the congressional debates preceding the passage of the 1986 Immigration Reform and Control Act, the last comprehensive immigration reform, frequently referred to as the 1986 Amnesty. She found a persistent preoccupation on the part of lawmakers (which was reflected in broader public discourses) about undocumented women's fecundity. They particularly feared that women would become pregnant during their process of legalization, thus upsetting the imagined aim of legalization: female immigrant workers applying for amnesty, tainted by their hyperfertility, would be replaced by idle and presumably indigent immigrant mothers and their children. Pease Chock writes: "These women who were 'illegal immigrants' would become legal residents, their children citizens, and both, 'public charges'" (1996, 2). She skillfully traces the historical association between (male) citizen-subjects, "an income-producing worker, one who is rational and orderly, one who is head of a nuclear family that replicates the qualities of its head—that is, a unit that is productive, self-sufficient, and

orderly," and (female) illegal aliens, "dependent, irrational or disorderly, unproductive and unpaid" (1).

In this way, illegal aliens are gendered as female and type-cast as public
charges, and thus their children are turned into unwanted and by necessity
dependent and disorderly public charges. Far from being seen as the progeni-
tors of a new generation of Americans, they serve instead as an unpleasant
reminder of the social and biological reproduction of abject undocumented and
deportable workers, reproduction that preferably occurs out of sight in distant
communities of immigrant-sending countries (Chang 2000; De Genova 2005;
Pease Chock 1996). Pierette Hondagneu-Sotelo and Ernestine Avila call this
expectation the "externalization of the costs of labor reproduction to Mexico
and Central America" (1997, 568; also De Genova 2009, 2005; Sider 2003).
Nicholas De Genova calls the relationship of the United States to undocumented immigrants a "constitutive contradiction": "The 'illegal' migrant's
ever-vexed placement within the juridical order of citizenship, while always by
definition outside of it, precisely as its most abject 'alien,'—her peculiar social
relation of juridical non-relationality—is the material and practical precondi-
tion for her thorough-going incorporation within a wider capitalist social
formation—as labor" (2009, 247). Thus, in these formulations, immigrant
women can be (tolerated, undocumented) workers or (abject, public-benefits-
consuming) mothers, not both.

Latina immigrant women, especially Mexican, and their fertility, have
become the favored symbol of anti-immigrant movements, their bodies becoming what Chavez calls "ground zero in a war of not just words but also public
policies and laws": "Biological reproduction of Latinas combines with their
social reproduction in the popular imagination to produce fears about Latino
population growth as a threat to the nation—that is, 'the American people,' as
conceived in demographic and racial/ethnic terms. This threat materialized not
merely because of Latino population growth but also because Latino babies
transgress the border between immigrants and citizens. It is here that the
metaphor of leaky national borders converges with that of porous bodies
(producing babies) and the permeable category of citizenship" (2008, 71–72).

In this way, although migration can sometimes hold certain emancipatory
features for women in the renegotiation of gender roles, work outside the home,
financial autonomy, and more (Hirsch 2003; Hondagneu-Sotelo 2003; Smith
2005), in other ways, some immigrant mothers experience greater subjectification in the United States than they ever did at home. Although poverty and
exclusions based on ethnicity, language, class, and other features were
described as frequent features of life for many Mexicans prior to migration,

there, at least, motherhood itself was at times a claim for agency (Browner 1986; Harvey et al. 2002; Martin 1990; Napolitano 2002, 166).

In the United States, Mexican immigrant women's babies are the opposite: justification for the denial of agency. Pregnancy, childbirth, and parenthood within the public health care system and their correlate, consumption of public benefits, are an entry into regimes of surveillance and subjectification that certainly do not erase but dramatically constrain women's agency and claims for citizenship (Piven and Cloward 1971, 17). Further, they make women eligible for vicious critiques within public discourse as "breeders," "baby machines," and mothers of "anchor," or "jackpot," babies. Even though progressive public institutions in largely immigrant-friendly places, like the hospital where I conducted research, can offer a degree of insulation from broad negative discourses, they are not completely immune from them. Nurses still laugh at patients leaving the maternity ward, teasing that they will see them soon. Women critique themselves and others for consuming too many resources. And most important, in this study, they eagerly rid themselves of the legacies of what they view as backward, even inhumane, reproductive care in their hometowns, hoping that their insertion into a modern, technologically sophisticated health care environment is the first sign that they are on their way to achieving the aspirations for which they migrated in the first place. The complicity of Mexican immigrant women in what amounts to a regime of subtractive health care may strip them of the protective features that enable them in the early years following their migration to have healthy, uncomplicated pregnancies. As these women become patients in the U.S. public health care system, they are also becoming citizens. It remains to be seen whether their patient pursuit of the rights and benefits of citizenship will be advanced or hindered by their insertion into the nation's public institutions.

Epilogue

As I complete this book, the Fourteenth Amendment of the U.S. Constitution is under attack. Legislators and activists at the state and federal levels are organizing to strategize ways to legislatively mandate a reinterpretation or revision of its guarantees of birth-right citizenship. The Fourteenth Amendment, adopted in the wake of the Civil War, in 1868, guaranteed equal protection under the law as well as birthright citizenship, a constitutional amendment deemed necessary because previously slaves and their descendants had been denied citizenship, a practice upheld by *Dred Scott v. Sandford* (1857). Advocates for revocation of the Fourteenth Amendment's guarantees cite some other nations' granting of citizenship based on *jus sanguinis*, citizenship by right of blood, or on lineage to citizens, versus *jus solis*, citizenship based on place of birth (see Knight 2005). They argue that citizenship should be granted only to the children of citizens, not on the basis of birth within the nation's borders. Jus sanguinis has been deeply criticized in some of the European states where it is law for allowing generations of people born in a country to never achieve the full rights of citizenship and also as a discriminatory process that reproduces ethnic homogeneity and defies contemporary pluralism.

Anxieties in the United States about porous borders and porous bodies have reached new heights. Immediately following the midterm elections in 2010, Republicans vowed to step up enforcement on the border and to introduce immigration-reform legislation, promising to use their House majority to reshuffle membership in the subcommittee on immigration (Martin 2010). The sum total of federal legislative efforts since the 2008 elections were a speech by President Barack Obama saying he looked forward to seeing immigration-reform legislation on his desk (with little reference to how that might occur) and a plan by Senate Majority Leader Harry Reid (D-NV) to bundle the defense-authorization bill with the DREAM Act, which would have allowed certain foreign-born, undocumented graduates of U.S. high schools to earn conditional permanent residency by meeting educational or military-service requirements, a plan that died before even coming up for debate. In the meantime, fueled by economic anxieties, Tea Party activism, and a rise in xenophobic popular discourse, state legislatures have been busily debating proposals to "fix" immigration law amid a purported federal unwillingness or inability to address immigration issues. The most renowned example of such legislation is SB 1070, the "Papers Please" law in Arizona, a punitive act allowing law-enforcement officials to proactively question the immigration status of individuals.

Receiving less of an uproar than SB1070 have been the multiple efforts by some of the same legislators, and others, to amend the constitutional guarantee of birthright citizenship for the children of undocumented immigrants. Russell Pearce, Republican state senator in Arizona, who proposed SB 1070 and also a bill to ban ethnic studies in the state, introduced in Arizona legislation that would deny state citizenship to the children of undocumented immigrants. Pearce belongs to a coalition of lawmakers, the Fourteenth Amendment Citizens Model Committee, who plan to introduce similar legislation in other states and also, were they to have the numbers of votes needed in the U.S. Congress, to call for a constitutional convention to repeal the Fourteenth Amendment at the federal level. This effort has been supported by, among others, Senator Lindsey Graham (R-SC), who said on cable television, "People come here to have babies, they come here to drop a child, it's called 'drop and leave'" (*Fox News*, July 29, 2010).

The Fourteenth Amendment, arguably, established national citizenship. Rather than "citizens," the Constitution refers to the "people" of the United States, and it has historically been interpreted to apply to all those living within the borders of the nation. Supreme Court precedent in *United States v. Wong Kim Ark* (1898) established that a child of foreign nationals (excluding diplomats stationed in the United States) enjoys birthright status as granted in the Fourteenth Amendment, irrespective of the citizenship of his or her parents, and *Plyler v. Doe* (1982) held that the children of undocumented immigrants are "persons" in "all ordinary senses of the term" and thus eligible for all the rights guaranteed by the Constitution.

It is unlikely that Pearce and his allies will be able to marshal the majority they need in both chambers of congress to consider a change to the Constitution, much less convoke the 75 percent of states they would need to call a constitutional convention, but it is increasingly clear that their efforts to gut the Fourteenth Amendment's guarantees of citizenship to all who are born in the United States do not require such measures. Instead, their hope is to legislate via litigation. By passing local and state laws that they are aware would be considered unconstitutional by virtually any legal scholar, these activists hope to provoke law suits that will not only generate heated debate but will face constitutional challenges that, if they achieve their goal, will be taken all the way to the Supreme Court. In this way, they wish to accelerate and manipulate the process of judicial review to set new legal precedent on the Fourteenth Amendment's guarantees. Their realistic hope is not to rewrite the Fourteenth Amendment but to change the way it has historically been interpreted to revoke long-standing guarantees of birthright citizenship.

The mere fact that these debates about the Fourteenth Amendment are occurring are evidence that the process of dehumanization of immigrants has reached new extremes. Deploying Giorgio Agamben's notion of "bare life," Nicholas De Genova argues that "if 'bare life' is the vanishing ground of the citizen in the state's disappearing act of 'sovereignty,' it is no less the foundational element of sovereign power that obstinately resurfaces in the figure of the non-citizen" (2009, 248).

The increasing ire about "anchor babies" and their parents is a symptom of the growing reality that the seemingly marginal figure of the undocumented immigrant is in fact at the heart of what the United States is today and will be tomorrow. The processes of "self-making and being-made by power relations" (Ong 1996, 738), like those described in this book—in which immigrant mothers simultaneously make gains in their own projects of superación and are schooled into what is expected of them by public agencies and individuals they encounter—will have weighty consequences for the future. If these processes continue to be subtractive and racializing, it is not immigrant families but those of us who receive them who are responsible for diluting the nation's identity and promise.

In 2006 Elmhurst Hospital in Queens, New York, declared, according to forecasts by the U.S. Census Bureau, that its staff had delivered the 300 millionth American. His name was Emanuel Plata, and he was the child of immigrant parents from Puebla, Mexico (Roberts 2006). Although hospitals around the country claimed to have delivered the auspicious infant, demographers held that, statistically, he was likely to be a Hispanic boy, born in the Southwest (Roberts 2006). Little Emanuel Plata, whether or not he was number 300 million, is a fitting emblem of the trends described in this book. Asked whether he felt lucky that his family had achieved such notoriety, his father reportedly replied, "My baby is healthy. My wife is fine. What more luck do I want?" (Roberts 2006). As various sectors of the United States debate the costs and benefits of immigration and the worthiness of undocumented immigrants for legalization, citizenship, benefits, and health care, Mexican immigrant parents like the Platas are frequently just trying to take care of their families. It is important that thought be given to the responsibility public institutions and private citizens have for facilitating their efforts.

Chapter 1 — Paradoxes and Patients: Immigrants and Prenatal Care

1. In contemporary American English, the word *chicken* is a catch-all term. However, in Spanish, and in many rural areas of Latin America, as in Marisol's hometown, *gallina, pollo,* and *gallo* (hen, chicken, and rooster) are very different terms, referring to both the age and the sex of the poultry in question. Caldo de gallina, made from a bird with a rangier flavor than younger chickens, is known to be especially fortifying. Serving caldo de gallina to pregnant women and women who have just given birth is a practice common in some parts of the Dominican Republic, Peru, Mexico, and surely elsewhere as well.

2. All these risk factors are questionable and problematical in various ways. To take only one example, "unmarried mother" refers to any woman who is not legally married. Although many of the women in this study were not married in the civil sense, only two of the study's participants were "single mothers," raising or planning to raise their child/ren on their own. When I asked women's civil status, many said *casada,* married, while others told me *juntada,* together, indicating a common-law relationship. There are various obstacles to legal marriage even for those couples who desire it in many parts of rural Mexico: costs (for the party, as well as for the officiant and license), the lack of a clerical presence in many rural hamlets, the migration of one of the partners, and more. In the United States, there are other barriers, including the documentation requirements of civil-marriage bureaus. Nonetheless, embarking on a life together, often marked by an elopement and pregnancy, is often considered to make the issue of the status of a couple's relationship moot. For the Department of Health and Mental Hygiene in New York City, however, *married* is a category defined narrowly in the legal sense.

3. This statistic may indicate that the department's efforts have not reached or have not affected Mexican immigrant women's birth outcomes, although they have been accompanied by dramatic improvements for other groups. It is also possible that department efforts have staved off a rise in rates of low birth weight and infant mortality or that the continued influx of new migrants has masked the worsening of birth outcomes of Mexican American women and immigrant women with greater duration in the United States. Further research is necessary to answer these questions.

4. I am grateful to Jennifer Hirsch and her colleagues at the Mailman School of Public Health at Columbia University, Virginia Raugh, Peter Messeri, and Joanne Csete, for their feedback on my project, particularly on this area.

5. This is an exceedingly specious argument with little empirical validity. In fact, a U.S.-citizen child has virtually no capacity to affect her undocumented parents' immigration status before reaching the age of twenty-one years. In addition, when undocumented parents are issued deportation orders, appeals based on the hardship caused to U.S.-citizen children are almost never successful (see Massey and Sánchez 2010).

6. George Marcus called for multisited ethnographic fieldwork in his seminal essay, "Ethnography in/of the World System": "[Multi-sited ethnography] claims that any

ethnography of a cultural formation in the world system is also an ethnography of the system, and therefore cannot be understood only in terms of the conventional single-site mise-en-scene of ethnographic research, assuming indeed it is the cultural formation, produced in several different locales, rather than the conditions of a particular set of subjects, that is the object of study" (1995, 99).

7. At the prenatal clinic, some women were accompanied by their partners; when they were, the men were invited to join in the interviews. Each time they took part, I also had the opportunity to interview the same women by themselves on another visit. At the community center, interviews were conducted weekday mornings. Women frequently said they were able to come to the center while their partners were at work and their school-age children were in school. When a spouse or children unexpectedly had the day off, a woman would typically not arrive. Thus, interviews at the community center were exclusively of women. Some interviews of women recruited through snowball methods occurred in their homes, but these too occurred at times of their choosing, which, typically, were weekdays while their spouse and children were out of the house.

8. Women recruited in other phases of the research, in the community center and through snowball methods, were interviewed in sites of their choosing. These phases fell under a protocol previously approved by an institutional review board.

9. One patient declined to participate following the consent procedure, and two women asked follow-up questions, but the rest agreed to participate upon completing the consent procedure.

10. Flyers about the study were posted in the prenatal clinic and given to physician's assistants, who distributed them to prenatal patients. In fact, this clinic served only women over the age of eighteen. Pregnant teens were served at another clinic to which I did not have access.

11. Although the number of births is reliable, the "per 1000" in these equations is trickier because it requires drawing on two incompatible data sources: the New York City Department of Health and Mental Hygiene's *Summary of Vital Statistics* and the U.S. Census. The *Summary of Vital Statistics* is presumably an accurate source of the number of total births to Mexican-nationality women in the city, but the total number of Mexican women ages 15–44 is not precisely known. The census estimates 289,755 Mexicans resided in New York State in 2007 (Bergad 2008), but this number may be low because New York has a low rate of census participation. In 2010, New York State broke records, with a 67 percent completion rate compared with 74 percent nationwide (U.S. Census Bureau 2010). Even though the census assumes a 1.9 percent undercount nationwide (U.S. Census Bureau 1990), the undercount for Hispanics, for New York City, and, in particular, for undocumented immigrants has historically been far higher, with estimates ranging from 5 to 20 percent (Duany 1992). Three of New York City's counties (Kings, Bronx, and New York) were among the five counties nationwide estimated to have the largest losses of federal funding because of census undercounts in 2000 (U.S. Census Monitoring Board 2001). Ethnic and mainstream media reported during the 2010 census a marked reluctance on the part of some immigrant groups to complete census forms, as well as various boycotts of the census promoted by grassroots organizations (Associated Press 2010; Correal 2010; Garett-Clark 2010). Further, Mexican immigrant women often initiate childbearing upon migration, skewing period estimates (Parrado and Valencia 2010, 2).

Chapter 2 — Immigrant Aspirations and the Decisions Families Make

1. See Alison Lee (2008) on this notion, which she calls "salir adelante."

2. *Coyote* and *pollero* refer to those who smuggle people across the U.S.-Mexican border for a fee. The fee ranges widely, depending on the client's nationality and how vulnerable or weak the client is perceived to be. Non-Mexicans are charged far higher rates than Mexicans, and women with infants and children, unaccompanied children, the elderly, sick, or disabled are charged higher rates. Although crossing typically involves walking through the desert, for a steep price some migrants contract to be taken across with false documents hidden in secret compartments in vehicles or, in the case of babies, carried across with someone else's baby's passport (Gálvez 2009; Hellman 2008).

3. Thank you to Jennifer Hirsch (personal communication) for suggesting this connection to the consumption of health care.

4. By most measures, New York City continues to be an "immigrant-friendly" city compared with most other places in the United States. With Mayor Michael Bloomberg's executive order 31, "Immigration Service Provider Law," prohibiting city employees from inquiring about the immigration status of anyone who seeks public services, his June 2010 statements in favor of immigration reform, and the city's refusal to participate in Section 287(g), part of the 1996 Illegal Immigration Reform and Immigrant Responsibility Act, which deputized police around the country to participate in enforcing federal immigration laws, the city has been derisively labeled a "sanctuary city" by some anti-immigrant organizations; but most immigrant advocates and immigrants would not go so far as to argue that it yet is.

5. Or, as Gregory Rodriguez phrases it, "mongrels, bastards, orphans, and vagabonds" (2008).

6. The Minuteman Project is described on its webpage as a "Multiethnic Immigration Law-Enforcement Advocacy Group: Operating Within the Law to Support Enforcement of the Law" (http://www.minutemanproject.com).

7. As of this writing, a judge had suspended some provisions of SB 1070 prior to their scheduled activation on July 29, 2010, but the state of Arizona was expected to appeal. Meanwhile, other states were busily debating similar legislative proposals, and some officials in Arizona appeared to be enforcing SB 1070 as it was written in spite of the judge's injunction.

8. Chavez (2009) discusses the construction of these discourses, but the last section of this paragraph was transmitted to me by members of the Minuteman Project protesting a day-laborer recruitment site outside a Home Depot store in San Diego, California, in August 2006. The group of which I was part, a bilingual, multinational, and multiethnic team of sociologists and anthropologists who were serving as neutral human-rights observers, were apparently taken for being Mexican, and elite at that, and told that we, as "Spaniards," were responsible for the lack of development of "our" country and that we should go back and make the country equitable so that the "poor Indians" did not have to migrate. "You're the racists!" they shouted at us. Although it took me time to make sense of this discourse, reading some of the restrictionist and nativist materials on internet at sites like vdare.com, minutemanproject.com, and americanpatrol.com helped me to decipher the arguments made by these groups.

9. This view is held even amid counter-interpretations like the fact that the United States has some of the fewest subsidized or affordable childcare options available to working families among industrialized nations (Chang 2000).

10. Jacoby notes that the easiest solution to the flow of unauthorized immigration is to double the number of available visas, thus bringing it into alignment with the number of jobs available and removing the incentive for unauthorized migration. (These figures precede the economic crisis that began in 2008.)

11. Here, I use "his" and "he" in acknowledgment of the fact that, historically, labor migration from Mexico has been predominantly male. Only since heightened border enforcement since 1990 have families decided to settle in the United States, and the numbers of women migrants have almost matched those of male migrants.

12. Of course, many workers do not make it to retirement. It has been estimated that one Mexican worker dies per day in the United States (Pritchard 2004), and many more are disabled and injured from working in the most dangerous jobs with few labor and safety protections.

13. Russell Pearce, who wrote Arizona's SB 1070, followed shortly thereafter, in June 2010, with a plan to make children born to undocumented immigrants in Arizona ineligible for U.S. citizenship, a direct assault on the jurisdiction of the United States Constitution to determine eligibility for citizenship. Arizona's Senator John Kyl (R) also has expressed support for a constitutional amendment revoking birthright citizenship for the children of undocumented immigrants (So 2010).

14. These confessions were made in a conversation with a former high-level Mexican diplomat who had been part of Mexico's team during the negotiation of NAFTA.

15. Hellman (2008) details these discussions.

16. I was told by a scholar of migration in Puebla, Mexico, that fees charged by coyotes for migrants from Puebla headed to New York City have risen to as much as $4,000 per person (Marcela Ibarra Mateos, personal communication, November 2010).

17. In 1994, seventy-nine scholars of poverty, labor markets, and family structures issued a press release stating that there was no evidence that women's childbearing decisions were linked to the availability of welfare (Sheldon Danziger, cited in Chang 2000).

18. Public school in Mexico is subsidized up to the sixth grade (Valenzuela 1999, 12).

19. When discussing this study with students in an undergraduate course, one student said, "I have nothing against Mexicans, but when I see a mom at a McDonald's with seven kids, I get upset." On such occasions, I have questioned whether one can assume that a woman seen in public is the mother of the children she accompanies. I told this student that the children may belong to neighbors or sisters, or the woman may be employed as a home daycare provider.

20. Undocumented men participate in the labor force at the rate of 94 percent, versus 85 percent for other immigrants and 83 percent for native-born men (Passel and Cohn 2009, 13).

Chapter 3 — Remembering Reproductive Care in Rural Mexico

1. A woman's husband's brother is her *cuñado;* her husband's brother's wife is her concuña. In other words, the two women are co-sisters-in-law. In this unusual case, Isabel's husband was Marta's cuñado and her *concuño,* her sister's husband and her husband's brother, as was Marta's husband for Isabel.

2. This is what I call the "McDonald's hypothesis," which is the first explanation many Mexican immigrants and others offered to me for the birth-weight paradox.

3. John Hoberman, in his critique of tropes of "primitive women," makes clear that Luisa's observation is not unique. He draws on mid-twentieth-century medical texts: "The easy labors of 'primitive women' are made possible by the simplicity of

their lives, while 'our present civilization with its artificial refinements and customs has made women less able nervously and physically to stand the strain of a hard, prolonged labor'" (Hoberman 2005, 95, quoted in Bridges 2011).

4. Barbara Kingsolver offers a nice rendition of these dynamics and the association of the United States with modernity and Mexico with tradition, albeit in a fictional form. Thank you to Jennifer Hirsch for recommending the book.

    [Mr. Shepherd:] "Why did Americans make off with the historical artifacts of Mexico to put them, where did he say? In the Peabody museum?"

    [Mrs. Brown:] "It's the same as your books, Mr. Shepherd. It's somebody else's gold pieces and bad luck. If we fill up our museums with that, we won't have to look at the dead folk lying at the bottom of our own water wells."

    "Who is *we*?"

    She pondered this, eyebrows lowered. "Just Americans," she said at length. "That's the only kind of person I know how to be. Not like you."

    "You'd do that? Take scissors and cut off your past?"

    "I did already. My family would tell you I went to the town and got above my raisings. It's what [my sister] calls 'modern.'"

    "And what would you call it?"

    "American. Like I said. The magazines tell us we're special. Not like the ones that birthed us. Brand-new. They paint a picture of some old-country rube with a shawl on her head, and make you fear you'll be like that, unless you buy cake mix and a home freezer."

    "But that sounds lonely. Walking around without any ancestors."

    "I don't say it's good. It's just how we be. I hate to say it, but that rube in the shawl is my sister, and I don't want to be her. I can't help it." (2010, 399)

5. Perhaps also for that reason learning to make kinship charts was not part of my anthropological training.

6. Smuggling infants across the border is one of the most lucrative specializations a coyote can have, and the techniques for doing so are elaborate, from specially built compartments in vehicles to using the passports of U.S.-born children. For families, arranging for children to cross the border is one of the riskiest and most costly migration endeavors; many families opt instead for prolonged separations, leaving children with relatives in Mexico (Dreby 2010; see also Hellman 2008).

7. This belief is supported by research, including work by Ellen Simpson and her colleagues (1994), in which women described fears that a fetus could be harmed if cravings were not indulged. One possible outcome was that a baby could be born with her mouth open, indicating the baby would have unsatisfied needs.

8. Simpson and her colleagues (2000) found that some women, fearful that soil is "dirty," seek to fulfill their craving to eat it by finding "clean dirt"; to indulge them magnesium carbonate blocks and small clay bricks stamped with the image of the Virgin of Guadalupe are sold in markets in California that cater to Mexican clientele.

9. Anthropologist Andrea Maldonado remarks (personal communication) that in Mexico City in 2010, the leftist government was also promoting "traditional" and "alternative" medicine in a variety of contexts. The district of Iztapalapa is the only district in Mexico City that promotes the teaching and practice of "traditional" medicine to its residents. Grassroots nongovernmental organizations, along with civil servants, are primarily responsible for these changes. Many social actors, including indigenous communities from all across Mexico, are also participating in these efforts.

10. Carole Browner gives a much more complex description of the reproductive issues for which medicinal plants are used in Oaxaca state than I am capable of providing here. She notes the use of plants for "speed[ing] and/or eas[ing] a birth, for postpartum recovery, excessive menstrual bleeding (menorrhagia), menstrual hemorrhaging, menstrual pain (dysmenorrhea), delayed menses, infertility, contraception, spontaneous abortion (miscarriage), and induced abortion" (1985, 484). She also offers a thorough inventory of the plants used in one part of the Sierra de Juárez and their applications.

11. Laurel and alcanfor may be from the same plant. Alcanfor is typically found as a solid waxy substance from the camphor laurel. Laurel is the term used for leaves that may be from the same plant or another genus.

12. Andrea Maldonado (personal communication) notes that in urban settings, too, temazcales have now been constructed, including one that accommodates one hundred people in Cerro de la Estrella Iztapalapa, Mexico City.

13. Historically, women in many cultures gave birth in a kneeling or squatting position; see Ricardo Jones (2009) and Janet Belaskas (1992) for descriptions of the process by which biomedical approaches replaced these practices with a rather more static, prostate birthing position. Edda Alatorre Wynter (1990) describes typical birthing postures, with kneeling predominant, in Central Mexico prior to the Conquest.

14. In anthropologist Valentina Napolitano's research, women from the countryside were more likely to be given a reprieve from work during and immediately after pregnancy than urban-dwelling women (2002, 166).

15. I was told by Tere that in some towns in Oaxaca in the contemporary period a family might offer their daughter in marriage in exchange for a cow.

16. As of this writing, thirteen Mexican pesos were the equivalent of one U.S. dollar.

17. The information contained in this section was gathered in an extended interview over two days in August 2008.

18. Gutmann, citing Sesia (1996), notes that midwifery is considered a subaltern practice to biomedical hegemony in Oaxaca and that many doctors responded to Oaxaca's Decree 345, mandating official accommodation of traditional medicine, with fear that it would turn the state into a laughing stock, that it would be seen as backward and would be characterized as the site of "Indian medicine" (2007, 190).

19. For a thorough historiography of the landscape of health care in Mexico, see Kaja Finkler (2004).

20. These processes are more complex and multivariate than what is implied in the quotation by Menéndez when viewed on a national scale with contradictory processes of incorporation and marginalization of practices denominated "traditional medicine" (Andrea Maldonado, personal communication).

21. Some, however, may view these requirements as an opportunity to increase the prestige of their office. Thank you to Andrea Maldonado for pointing this possibility out.

22. The rate actually dropped to 29.9 in 1997, but rose again ten points, in part because of a change in the criteria for classifying maternal mortality.

23. Oportunidades gained some notoriety in New York City when Mayor Bloomberg and a task force studied its cash pay-outs to families for well-child visits, immunizations, and so on, for possible replication in the city (World Bank 2008).

Chapter 4 — Becoming Patients: Birth Experiences in New York City

1. Although my research was not focused on comparisons between Mexicans and other groups, in the course of research I was able to notice that attitudes among hospital personnel about Mexican patients and their attitudes toward other patients were

sometimes starkly different. When I described the topic of my research, the midwives and some of the doctors were encouraging and offered their own hypotheses: it's the diet, it's the way that Mexican families rally around a pregnant woman, they are healthy, they welcome every pregnancy. The patients who were subjected to the most overtly disparaging discussion among physician's assistants were women dressed in Muslim head and body coverings. I heard physician's assistants say in front of patients (1) that they were all beaten by their husbands, (2) that the husbands say they are here to translate but they are here to control their wives and make sure they do not get birth control or sterilization, (3) that they did not trust the women or their husbands. This attitude extended even outside the hospital: a few medical assistants said that in the past they patronized a deli across the street from the hospital, but after the deli owner brought his wife for prenatal care and they saw she covered her head, they decided not to shop in his store.

2. One in three births in the United States is covered by Medicaid (Conley, Strully, and Bennet 2003, 126).

3. It is important to note that, apart from my research on the topic, having given birth to the first of my own children with an obstetrician and the second with a midwife, my subjective experiences convinced me of the superiority of a midwifery approach in uncomplicated pregnancies and deliveries.

4. In my research practice, I subscribe to an anthropological ethics that asserts the importance of taking the side of those among whom one conducts research as a necessary point of departure (Hymes 1972; see van der Geest and Finkler, 2004, on hospital ethnography). Although anthropology concerned with studying individuals within institutions and studying "up" has complicated this simple ethics, I nevertheless feel that even within institution-based research one must have a basic respect for the mission and premise of the institution and the individuals who work within or are served by it. It would be methodologically easy and also theoretically facile to find a public institution that mistreats its clients and to focus on that mistreatment. As a scholar of immigration, I am aware that it is not difficult to find institutions that exclude and mistreat immigrants, especially undocumented ones. However, I found it more urgent to conduct research into the ways that well-intentioned, well-functioning—if beleaguered—institutions and their staff, clients, funders, and more sometimes miss the mark, misunderstand each other, and reproduce inequalities. Although I might have situated my research in one of the several hospitals about which women told me horror stories of mistreatment, I felt it was more productive to place myself in a public hospital that has made earnest and considered efforts to reach out to and serve immigrant patients with respect and superior care. In such a setting, my critiques of the shortcomings of that care and suggestions for its improvement might be heard and even implemented.

5. In her speech, Annette uses unconventional colloquial terms. For example, *cualificas* is incorrect; the correct verb is *calificar*. Also, when Annette asks, "No coges cupones?" both the verb *coger* and the noun *cupones* are not standard. Coger is used only in some parts of the Spanish-speaking world for getting or taking (and in other places, including Mexico, it can be a vulgar term for sexual intercourse). Food stamps, in standard Spanish, is *cupones de alimentos*; the word *cupón* alone has a variety of different meanings; thus, the word can be confusing to someone not familiar with the terms for the various kinds of public assistance.

Although Annette, a New York–born woman of Puerto Rican descent, told me Spanish is her first language, her use of nonstandard terms was illustrative of the ways that potential misunderstandings go beyond simple issues of the accessibility of translation and Spanish-speaking personnel. Although translation is mandated in city hospitals, qualified, trained translators are not always available. and there is often an assumption that those who self-identify as or are presumed to be "Spanish speakers" can adequately serve Spanish-dominant patients (see Siulc 2003). At Manhattan Hospital, translators were available on a phone installed in every room where patients were attended, but I never observed anyone use the phone to obtain translation for Spanish-speaking patients.

When Annette told Carmen she would qualify for more aid when the baby was born, she implicitly acknowledged that she was probably aware of Carmen's undocumented immigration status, even though, in keeping with New York City's Executive Order 41, she did not ask Carmen her status directly. An undocumented mother cannot qualify for anything more than emergency Medicaid and WIC through the PCAP program and is ineligible for food stamps.

6. Some women made inferences about or, in one case, explicitly told me stories of rape during border crossing.

7. However, aspects of pregnancy care as seemingly objective as recommended glucose levels vary significantly. The American Diabetic Association and the American College of Obstetricians and Gynecologists recommend glucose levels lower than those used to diagnose gestational diabetes, or diabetes mellitus, in some European countries; thus more women are diagnosed with gestational diabetes in the United States and are referred to high-risk clinics.

8. Some quotations are written in English. In some of the participant-observation portions of the research for this book, I did not audio-record interactions but reproduced them from notes taken at the time or shortly thereafter. Because I did not note down wording verbatim, I represent these conversations in the language in which I wrote them down.

9. As mentioned in Chapter 1, my research methodologies did not enable me to follow most patients into the labor and delivery ward. I relied on them to contact me if they wished for me to be present. Although many women said they would, citing my ability to translate and to explain interactions with providers, for women to retain my phone number and think to call me when the time came was not easy.

10. Douglas Massey and Magaly Sánchez also relate respondents' experiences with differential treatment at the hands of Spanish-speaking medical personnel, especially Puerto Ricans (2010, 133), as does Nina Siulc (2003). This is an important area for additional research.

11. *Muchacha* is the term also used to refer to a female domestic servant.

12. In fact, my younger son's car seat was used by more than one family for this purpose.

13. Even though I visited Diana at her apartment after her child was born, I did not learn whether she eventually obtained a crib.

Chapter 5 — Critical Perspectives on Prenatal Care

1. Elya told me that she tended to be quick to anger, but that during pregnancy she tried to remain calm because people had told her that her baby would cry a lot if she spent a lot of time angry during pregnancy.

2. None of the women interviewed reported drug use before, during, or after pregnancy.

3. *Aliviarse*, to alleviate oneself, is the verb most participants in this study used for "to give birth." But *aliviarse* may be commonly used only in Mexico; the most standard Spanish translation is *dar a luz*, to give or bring to light.

4. This discouragement of working may be different from when a male partner discourages or prohibits a female partner from working at all, which Marie Harvey and her colleagues find is more likely to be an exertion of male authority than a sign of benevolence (2002, 288).

5. This saying includes a play on words: the verb *casarse*, to marry (in this case, *casa, marries*), and the word for house, *casa*, sound the same and heighten the association in this saying between marriage and neolocal residence. This is an idea that is valued, even though neolocality may be delayed for years or decades or may involve constructing a new home on family-owned property. Julia Pauli renders this phrase as "la casada casa quiere" [a woman who marries wants a house] (2008, 178), and Hirsch, "la que se casa quiere casa" [she who marries wants a house]" (2003, 67).

6. "Crowding" has become one of the most controversial fronts for conflicts between those who would restrict immigration and immigration advocates. Many towns and cities across the United States have passed ordinances attempting to limit the number of members a "nuclear" family can include or to define how many people can reside in a dwelling designated "single-family." Increased vigilance and persecution of subdivision of housing units is one way in which those who rent to immigrants and immigrants themselves are exposed to state surveillance and sometimes harassment, ostensibly amidst concerns about public safety (Belson and Capuzzo 2007; Caldwell 2006). See Conley Strully, and Bennet on the negative correlation between crowding and low birth weight (2003, 70).

7. Many women in the study recounted being told by housemates that they were pregnant because of the color of their face, dark circles under their eyes, sleepiness, fatigue, and other clues.

8. Both these terms are identical cognates in Spanish and English. See Andrea Maldonado (2010a) for an extensive analysis of the construction of "normality" in Mexico with relevance to my discussion of the aspirational stance of Mexican immigrants in the United States.

9. Khiara Bridges (2011) suggests that women of color, who are perceived as stoic and with a high pain threshold. may be denied pain relief more often than white women under the assumption that they do not experience pain in the same way or as severely.

10. Karen's insistence is in keeping with recent developments in biomedical care. In July 2010, the American College of Obstetricians and Gynecologists relaxed its policy on VBAC delivery, stating that it "is a safe and appropriate choice for most women who have had a prior cesarean delivery, including for some women who have had two previous cesareans" (Steinweg 2010).

11. Reanne Frank and R. A. Hummer (2002) found that migration is correlated with favorable birth outcomes even for those who do not migrate: infants born in households in Mexico with members who have migrated are less likely to have low birth weights than infants in nonmigrant households.

12. At Manhattan Hospital, also, when women were called with results of their pregnancy test, they were asked whether they planned to continue with their pregnancies and were scheduled for an appointment corresponding to their answer: in the obstetric clinic or the gynecological clinic. Although this question was surely framed in a neutral fashion and as a routine part of the hospital's efforts to uphold its patients' reproductive freedom, some of the patients I interviewed reported being offended by the question, and a few interpreted it to carry an implication that providers thought their fetus should be aborted.

Chapter 6 — Prenatal Care and the Reception of Immigrants: Reflections and Suggestions for Change

1. In an off-the-record conversation with the author, a former Mexican foreign minister said that in negotiations surrounding NAFTA the predicted displacement of a half million peasants was considered a necessary human cost for the development of the nation and the liberalization of trade. In other contexts, another former foreign minister has said that Mexico put migration on the table of negotiations with NAFTA—circulation of goods, capital, *and* people—but that the United States limited discussions to only goods and capital. It is arguable that the failure of the signatories of NAFTA to liberalize the circulation of workers along with the flows of capital and goods is a key reason for the massive increase of unauthorized migration following the accord's implementation, even amid increased border militarization (Chang 2000; De Genova 2005; Gálvez 2009; Holmes 2009).
2. See Matthew Gutmann (2002, xxvi–xxvii), Nestor García Canclini (1982, 1993), and Guillermo Bonfil Batalla (1987) for more on the use of the term *clases populares* in Mexico.
3. *Inyección* is the term for birth control injections like Depo-Provera; *T de cobre* is the term frequently used for an intrauterine device.
4. However, one woman, Diana, had a lapse in her prenatal care between her fifteenth and twenty-ninth weeks. She had been visiting the hospital regularly for scheduled ultrasounds but had not been told that prenatal care and radiology were in two different areas and appointments for them were scheduled on two different calendars. Therefore, she attended only her ultrasound appointments. She was scolded when the error was finally discovered, even though anyone in radiology looking at her chart might have noticed that she had not visited the prenatal clinic for more than three months and inquired as to why.
5. For other health indicators, such as obesity, diabetes, hypertension, and heart disease, data have shown that within a few years of migrating Latino immigrants begin to show a decline in health advantages. For example, within five years of migrating, they are one and a half times more likely to have high blood pressure than they did when they first arrived (Centers for Disease Control data cited in *Unnatural Causes* 2007; see also Taningco 2007).

References

Abraído-Lanza, Ana F., A. N. Armbrister, K. R. Flórez, and A. N. Aguirre. 2006. "Toward a theory-driven model of acculturation in public health research." *American Journal of Public Health* 96(8):1342–1346.

Abraído-Lanza, Ana F., M. T. Chao, and K. R. Flórez. 2005. "Do healthy behaviors decline with greater acculturation? Implications for the Latino mortality paradox." *Social Science & Medicine* 61:1243–1255.

Abraído-Lanza, Ana F., Bruce Dohrenwend, Daisy Ng-Mak, and J. Blake-Turner. 1999. "The Latino mortality paradox: A test of the 'salmon bias' and healthy migrant hypotheses." *American Journal of Public Health* 89(10):1543–1548.

Access Denied Blog. 2009. "Access denied: A conversation on unauthorized immigration and health." http://accessdeniedblog.wordpress.com/.

Alatorre Wynter, Edda. 1990. "Atención a la salud en la sociedad novohispana: Origen de la enfermería." *Revista de Enfermería*, Instituto Mexicano del Seguro Social (México) 3(2/3):75–77.

———. 1994. "El Surgimiento de la enfermería professional en México. Reflexciones sobre su carácter femenino." *Revista de Enfermería*, Instituto Mexicano del Seguro Social (México) 6(1):47–51.

Alegría, Margarita, Glorisa Canino, Patrick Shrout, Meghan Woo, Naihua Duan, Doryliz Vila, María Torres, Chih-nan Checn, and Xiao-Li Meung. 2008. "Prevalence of mental illness in immigrant and non-immigrant U.S. Latino groups." *American Journal of Psychiatry* 165(3):359–369.

Alegría, Margarita, William Sribney, Meghan Woo, Maria Torres, and Peter Guarnaccia. 2007. "Looking beyond nativity: The relation of age of immigration, length of residence, and birth cohorts to the risk of onset of psychiatric disorders for Latinos." *Research on Human Development* 4(1):19–47.

Allday, Erin. 2007. "Fewer options for those who seek natural births: Midwives becoming less popular as cesarean sections gain ground." *San Francisco Chronicle*, May 29.

Alvarado, Virginia. 2010."The Mixteca people: Abandoned." *Diario de México*, March 29. In *Voices That Must Be Heard,* Edition 418, April 8. Translated by Emily Leavitt. http://www.indypressny.org/nycma/voices/418/.

American Academy of Pediatrics. 2005. "The changing concept of Sudden Infant Death Syndrome: Diagnostic coding shifts, controversies regarding the sleeping environment, and new variables to consider in reducing risk." *Pediatrics* 116(5): 1245–1255.

Appadurai, Arjun. 1996. *Modernity at Large: Cultural Dimensions of Globalization.* Minneapolis: University of Minnesota Press.

Associated Press. 2010. "US census on track but toughest part yet to come." *WAOW Wisconsin*, vol. 9. April 7. http://www.waow.com/global/story.asp?s=12275466.

Baer, Hans. 2001. *Biomedicine and Alternative Healing Systems in America: Issues of Class, Race, Ethnicity, and Gender.* Madison: University of Wisconsin Press.

———. 2004. *Toward an Integrative Medicine: Alternative Therapies Meet Biomedicine.* Walnut Creek, CA: Alta Mira Press.

Begier, Elizabeth, Regina Zimmerman, Stephen Schwartz, Kevin Koshar, Wenhui Li, Flor Betancourt, Tara Das, Ann Madsen. 2010. *Summary of Vital Statistics 2008.* http://www.nyc.gov/html/doh/downloads/pdf/vs/2008sum.pdf.

Belaskas, Janet. 1992. *Active Birth: The New Approach to Giving Birth Naturally.* Cambridge, MA: Harvard Common Press.

Belson, Ken, and Jill Capuzzo. 2007. "Towns rethink laws against illegal immigrants." *New York Times*, September 26.

Bergad, Laird. 2008. "Mexicans in New York City, 2007: An update." Latino Data Project, Report 26. http://web.gc.cuny.edu/lastudies/latinodataprojectreports/Mexicans%20in% 20New%20York%20City,%202007%20An%20Update.pdf.

———. 2009. "Distribution of the Mexican population of New York City by borough and foreign born." Personal communication.

Besserer, Federico, and Daniela Oliver. 2010. "Etnografía especular: Una contribución desde los estudios sobre la ciudad transnacional a las nuevas orientaciones en la etnografía." Unpublished manuscript, August 13.

Bickel, Alexander. 1975. *The Morality of Consent.* New Haven, CT: Yale University Press.

Biehl, João. 2005. *Vita: Life in a Zone of Social Abandonment.* Berkeley: University of California Press.

Bloomberg, Michael R. 2010. Weekly radio address, July 4. http://nyc.gov/portal/site/ nycgov/menuitem.c0935b9a57bb4ef3daf2f1c701c789a0/index.jsp?pageID=mayor_ press_release&catID=1194&doc_name=http%3A%2F%2Fnyc.gov%2Fhtml%2Fom %2Fhtml%2F2010b%2Fpr300–10.html&cc=unused1978&rc=1194&ndi=1.

Bonfil Batalla, Guillermo. 1987. *México Profundo.* México City: Grijalbo.

Borrell, Luisa. 2005. "Racial identity among Hispanics: Implications for health and well-being." *American Journal of Public Health* 95(3):379–381.

Bridges, Khiara. 2008. "Wily patients, welfare queens, and the racialization of pregnancy in a New York City obstetrics clinic." Paper presented at the meetings of the Society for Applied Anthropology/Society for Medical Anthropology, Memphis, Tennessee, March 27.

———. 2011. *Reproducing Race: An Ethnography of Pregnancy as a Site of Racialization.* Berkeley: University of California Press.

Briggs, Laura. 2002. *Reproducing Empire: Race, Sex, Science, and U.S. Imperialism in Puerto Rico.* Berkeley: University of California Press.

Browner, Carole. 1985. "Plants used for reproductive health in Oaxaca, México." *Economic Botany* 39(4):482–504.

———. 1986. "The politics of reproduction in a Mexican village." *Signs* 11(4):710–724.

———. 2000. "Situating women's reproductive activities." *American Anthropologist* 102(4):773–788.

Browner, Carole, and Sondra Perdue. 1988. "Women's secrets: Bases for reproductive and social autonomy in a Mexican community." *American Ethnologist* 15(1):84–97.

Browner, Carole, and Nancy Press. 1996. "The production of authoritative knowledge in American prenatal care." *Medical Anthropology Quarterly* 10(2):141–156.

Buekens, P., F. Notzon, M. Kotelchuck, and A. Wilcox. 2000. "Why do Mexican Americans give birth to few low-birth-weight infants?" *American Journal of Epidemiology* 152:347–351.

Caldwell, Christopher. 2006. "A family or a crowd?" *New York Times*, February 26.

Castro, Roberto. 2002. *La Vida en la Adversidad: El Significado de la Salud y la Reproducción en la Pobreza.* México City: Centro Regional de Investigaciones Multidisciplinarias.

Centers for Disease Control. 2009. "Births: Final Data for 2006," *National Vital Statistics Reports* 57(7). http://www.cdc.gov/nchs/data/nvsr/nvsr57/nvsr57_07.pdf.

Chang, Grace. 2000. *Disposable Domestics: Immigrant Women Workers in the Global Economy.* Boston: South End Press.

Chavez, Leo R. 1988. "Settlers and sojourners: The case of Mexicans in the United States." *Human Organization* 47(2):95–108.

———. 1997. "Immigration reform and nativism: The nationalist response to the transnationalist challenge." In *Immigrants Out! The New Nativism and the Anti-Immigrant Impulse in the United States,* edited by Juan Perea, 61–77. New York: New York University Press.

———. 2008. *The Latino Threat: Constructing Immigrants, Citizens, and the Nation.* Palo Alto, CA: Stanford University Press.

———. 2009. "The Latino threat and media constructions of nation." Plenary lecture presented at the Undocumented Hispanic Migration conference, Connecticut College, New London, Connecticut, October 16.

Cobas, José, Hector Balcazar, Mary Benin, Verna Keith, and Yinong Chong. 1996. "Acculturation and low-birth-weight infants among Latino women: A reanalysis of HHANES data with structural equation models." *American Journal of Public Health* 86(3):394–396.

Conley, Dalton, Kate Strully, and Neil Bennet. 2003. *Starting Gate: Birth Weight and Life Chances.* Berkeley: University of California Press.

Cook, B., M. Alegría, J. Y. Lin, and J. Guo. 2009. "Pathways and correlates connecting Latinos' mental health with exposure to the United States." *American Journal of Public Health* 99(12):2247–2254.

Correal, Annie. 2010. "Brooklyn neighborhoods receive fewer federal funds because of low level participation." *Carib News,* March 10. In *Voices That Must Be Heard,* Edition 415, March 17. Translated from the Spanish by Chris Brandt. http://www.indypressny.org/nycma/voices/415/news_1/news/.

Cortes, Sergio. 2003. "Migrants from Puebla in the 1990s." In *Immigrants and Schooling: Mexicans in New York,* edited by Regina Cortina, 183–204. Staten Island, NY: Center for Migration Studies.

Cosminsky, S. 1982. "Knowledge and body concepts of Guatemalan midwives." In *Anthropology of Human Birth,* edited by M. Kay, 233–252. Philadelphia: Davis.

Coutin, Susan Bibler. 2003. "Suspension of deportation hearings and measures of 'Americanness.'" *Journal of Latin American Anthropology* 8(2):58–95.

Cramer, James. 1987. "Social factors and infant mortality: Identifying high-risk groups and proximate causes." *Demography* 24(3):299–322.

Dávila, Arlene. 2008. *Latino Spin: Public Image and the Whitewashing of Race.* New York: New York University Press.

Davis-Floyd, Robbie. 1992. *Birth as an American Rite of Passage.* Berkeley: University of California Press.

———. 2001. "La partera profesional: Articulating identity and cultural space for a new kind of midwife in México." *Medical Anthropology* 20(2/3):4.

Davis-Floyd, Robbie, Lesley Barclay, Betty-Anne Daviss, and Jan Tritten, eds. 2009. *Birth Models That Work.* Berkeley: University of California Press.

Davis-Floyd, Robbie, and Elizabeth Davis. 1996. "Intuition as authoritative knowledge in midwifery and homebirth." *Medical Anthropology Quarterly* 10(2):237–269.

Davis-Floyd, Robbie, and Carolyn F. Sargent. 1996. "The social production of authoritative knowledge in pregnancy and childbirth." *Medical Anthropology Quarterly* 10(2):111–120.

————. 1997. *Childbirth and Authoritative Knowledge: Cross-Cultural Perspectives.* Berkeley: University of California Press.

De Genova, Nicholas. 2005. *Working the Boundaries: Race, Space and 'Illegality' in Mexican Chicago.* Durham, NC: Duke University Press.

————. 2009. "Sovereign power and the bare life of Elvira Arellano." *Feminist Media Studies* 9(2):245–250.

De Genova, Nicholas, and Ana Y. Ramos-Zayas. 2003. *Latino Crossings: Mexicans, Puerto Ricans, and the Politics of Race and Citizenship.* New York: Routledge.

Declercq, Eugene. 2009. "Births attended by certified nurse-midwives in the United States in 2005." *Journal of Midwifery and Women's Health* 1(9):95–96.

Devries, Raymond. 2004. "The trap of legal recognition." In *Midwifery and the Medicalization of Childbirth: Comparative Perspectives*, edited by Edwin R. Van Teijlingen, George W. Lowis, and Peter McCaffery, 209–318. Hauppage, NY: Nova Science Publishers.

Douglas, Mary. 1985. *Risk Acceptability According to the Social Sciences.* New York and London: Russell Sage/Routledge.

————. 1992. *Risk and Blame: Essays in Cultural Theory.* London and New York: Routledge.

Douglas, Mary, and A. Wildavsky. 1982. *Risk and Culture: An Essay on the Selection of Environmental and Technological Dangers.* Berkeley: University of California Press.

Dreby, Joanna. 2010. *Divided by Borders: Mexican Migrants and Their Children.* Berkeley: University of California Press.

Duany, Jorge. 1992. "The census undercount, the underground economy, and undocumented migration: The case of Dominicans in Santurce, Puerto Rico." http://www.census.gov/srd/papers/pdf/ev92–17.pdf.

Durand, Jorge. 2004. "From traitors to heroes: 100 years of Mexican migration policies." *Migration Information Source*, March. http://www.migrationinformation.org/feature/display.cfm?ID=203.

Eckersley, Richard. 2006. "Is modern Western culture a health hazard?" *International Journal of Epidemiology* 35(2):252–258.

Epstein, Abby. 2008. *The Business of Being Born.* Documentary film. Barranca Productions.

Escobar, J. I., and W. A. Vega. 2006. "Cultural issues and psychiatric diagnosis: Providing a general background for considering substance use diagnoses." *Addiction* 101:40–47.

Eunice Kennedy Shriver National Institute of Child Health and Human Development, National Institutes of Health, Department of Health and Human Services. 2005. *Safe Sleep for Your Baby: Reduce the Risk of Sudden Infant Death Syndrome (SIDS)—General Outreach.* Washington, DC: U.S. Government Printing Office.

Farmer, Paul. 2003. *Pathologies of Power: Health, Human Rights, and the New War on the Poor.* Berkeley: University of California Press.

Federation for American Immigration Reform. 2009. "Anchor babies: Part of the immigration-related American lexicon." http://www.fairus.org/site/PageServer?pagename=iic_immigrationissuecenters4608.

Feldhusen, Adrian. 2000. "The history of midwifery and childbirth in America: A timeline." *Midwifery Today.* http://www.midwiferytoday.com/articles/timeline.asp.

Fernández, Leticia, and Alison Newby. 2010. "Family support and pregnancy behavior among women in two Mexican border cities." *Frontera Norte* 22(43):7–34.

Fernández, Valeria. 2010. "Immigrant mothers in Arizona: Some vow to stay despite new law, others consider moving." *Feet in 2 Worlds.* http://news.feetintwoworlds.org/2010/05/14/immigrant-mothers-in-arizona-some-vow-to-stay-despite-new-law-others-consider-moving/.

Finkler, Kaja. 1994. "Sacred healing and biomedicine compared." *Medical Anthropology Quarterly* 8(2):178–197.

———. 2004. "Biomedicine globalized and localized: Western medical practices in an outpatient clinic of a Mexican hospital." *Social Science & Medicine* 59(10): 2037–2051.

Forbes, Douglas, and Parker Frisbie. 1991. "Spanish surname and Anglo infant mortality: Differentials over a half-century." *Demography* 28(4):639–660.

Foucault, Michel. 1988. "Technologies of the self." In *Technologies of the Self: A Seminar with Michel Foucault*, edited by L. H. Martin, 16–49. London: Tavistock.

———. 1991. "Governmentality." Translated by Rosi Braidotti and revised by Colin Gordon. In *The Foucault Effect: Studies in Governmentality*, edited by Graham Burchell, Colin Gordon, and Peter Miller, 87–104. Chicago: University of Chicago Press, 1991.

Frank, Reanne, and R. A. Hummer. 2002. "The other side of the paradox: The risk of low birth weight among infants of migrant and nonmigrant households within Mexico." *International Migration Review* 36(3):746–765.

Fuller, Bruce, Margaret Bridges, Edward Bein, Heeju Jang, Sunuong Jung, Sophia Rabe-Hesketh, Neal Huldon, and Alice Kun. 2009. "The health and cognitive growth of Latino toddlers: At risk or immigrant paradox?" *Maternal and Child Health Journal* 13(6):755–768.

Gálvez, Alyshia. 2009. *Guadalupe in New York: Devotion and the Struggle for Citizenship Rights among Mexican Immigrants*. New York and London: New York University Press.

———. 2010. "Resolviendo: How September 11th tested and transformed a New York City Mexican immigrant organization." In *Politics and Partnerships: The Role of Voluntary Associations in America's Political Past and Present*, edited by Elisabeth Clemens and Doug Guthrie, 297–326. Chicago: University of Chicago Press.

García Canclini, Nestor. 1982. *Las culturas populares en el capitalismo*. México City: Nueva Imagen.

———. 1993. *Transforming Modernity: Popular Culture in México*. Translated by Lidia Lozano. Austin: University of Texas Press.

Garrett-Clark, Andrew. 2010. "Overcoming fear of the 2010 Census." *Manhattan Times*, March 17. In *Voices That Must be Heard*, Edition 417, April 1. http://www .indypressny.org/nycma/voices/417/news/news.

Gaskin, Ina May. 2003. *Ina May's Guide to Childbirth*. New York: Bantam Books.

Gergen, Kenneth. 1994. *Realities and Relationships: Soundings in Social Construction*. Cambridge, MA: Harvard University Press.

Geronimus, Arline T. 1992. "The weathering hypothesis and the health of African-American women and infants: Evidence and speculations." *Ethnicity and Disease* (2):207–221.

Ginsburg, Faye, and Rayna Rapp. 1995. *Conceiving the New World Order: The Global Politics of Reproduction*. Berkeley: University of California Press.

Glick-Schiller, Nina. 1992. "What's wrong with this picture? The hegemonic construction of culture in AIDS research in the United States." *Medical Anthropology* 6(3):237–254.

Gobierno del Estado de Oaxaca. 2009. Accessed November 23, 2009. http://www.oaxaca .gob.mx/.

Goer, Henci. 1995. *Obstetric Myths versus Research Realities*. Westport, CT: Bergin & Garvey.

González, Nancie. 1986. "Giving birth in America: The immigrant dilemma." In *International Migration: The Female Experience,* edited by Rita James Simon and Caroline Brettell, 241–253. Totowa, NJ: Rowman & Allenheld.

Griswold, Daniel. 2009. "As immigrants move in, Americans move up." *Cato Institute Free Trade Bulletin,* July 21.

Guarnaccia, Peter, and Orlando Rodríguez. 1996. "Concepts of culture and their role in the development of culturally competent mental health services." *Hispanic Journal of Behavioral Sciences* 18(4):419–443.

Guarnaccia, Peter, Teresa Vivar, Anne C. Bellows, and Gabriela Alcaraz. 2010. "'We eat meat every day': Ecology and economy of dietary change among Oaxacan migrants from Mexico to New Jersey." Unpublished manuscript.

Guendelman, Sylvia, and Barbara Abrams. 1995. "Dietary intake among Mexican-American women: Generational differences and a comparison with white non-Hispanic women." *American Journal of Public Health* 85(1):20–25.

Gutiérrez, Elena. 2008. *Fertile Matters: The Politics of Mexican-Origin Women's Reproduction.* Austin: University of Texas Press.

Gutmann, Matthew. 1996. *The Meanings of Macho.* Berkeley: University of California Press.

———. 2002. *The Romance of Democracy: Compliant Defiance in Contemporary México.* Berkeley: University of California Press.

———. 2007. *Fixing Men: Sex, Birth Control, and AIDS in México.* Berkeley: University of California Press.

Harley, Kim G. 2004. "Examining an epidemiological paradox: The role of acculturation, nutrition, and social support in the birth outcomes of women of Mexican descent." PhD diss., University of California at Berkeley.

Harvey, S. Marie, Linda J. Beckman, Carole H. Browner, and Christy A. Sherman. 2002. "Relationship power, decision making, and sexual relations: An exploratory study with couples of Mexican origin." *Journal of Sex Research* 39(4):284–291.

Hayes-Bautista, D. E. 2002. "The Latino health agenda for the twenty-first century." In *Latinos: Remaking America,* edited by M. Suárez-Orozco and M. Páez, 215–235. Berkeley: University of California Press.

Hays, Bethany. 1996. "Authority and authoritative knowledge in American birth." *Medical Anthropology Quarterly* 10(2):291–294.

Hellman, Judith Adler. 1995. *Mexican Lives.* New York: New Press.

———. 2008. *The World of Mexican Migrants: Between the Rock and the Hard Place.* New York: New Press.

———. 2009. "To stay or return home? New factors shaping the decisions of undocumented Mexican migrants." Plenary lecture, given at the Undocumented Hispanic Migration conference, Connecticut College, New London, Connecticut, October 16.

Hessol, N. A., and E. Fuentes-Afflick. 2000. "The perinatal advantage of Mexican-origin Latina women." *Annals of Epidemiology* 10:516–523.

Hirsch, Jennifer. 2003. *A Courtship after Marriage: Sexuality and Love in Mexican Transnational Families.* Berkeley: University of California Press.

Hirsch, Jennifer, Holly Wardlow, Daniel Jordan Smith, Harriet M. Phinney, Shanti Parikh, and Constance A. Nathanson. 2010. *The Secret: Love, Marriage, and HIV.* Nashville, TN: Vanderbilt University Press.

Hoberman, John. 2005. "The primitive pelvis: The role of racial folklore in obstetrics and gynecology during the twentieth century." In *Body Parts: Critical Explorations in*

Corporeality, edited by Christopher E. Forth and Ivan Crozier, 85–104. Lanham, MD: Lexington Books.

Hoffman, Beatrix. 2006. "Sympathy and exclusion: Access to health care for undocumented immigrants in the United States." In *A Death Retold: Jesica Santillán, the Bungled Transplant, and Paradoxes of Medical Citizenship*, edited by Keith Wailoo, Julie Livingston, and Peter Gaurnaccia, 237–254. Chapel Hill: University of North Carolina Press.

Hoffman, Jan. 2005. "A Conversation with Janet Golden: Sorting out ambivalence over alcohol and pregnancy." *New York Times*, Health, January 25.

Holmes, Seth. 2009. "Strawberries, suffering, and symbolic violence: Health policy debates and public representations of undocumented indigenous Mexican migrants in the United States." Paper presented at the annual meeting of the American Anthropological Association, Philadelphia. December 3.

Hondagneu-Sotelo, Pierette. 1995. "Beyond 'the longer they stay' (and say they will stay): Women and Mexican immigrant settlement." *Qualitative Sociology* 18(1):21–43.

Hondagneu-Sotelo, Pierette, ed. 2003. *Gender and U.S. Immigration: Contemporary Trends*. Berkeley: University of California Press.

———. (2001) 2007. *Doméstica: Immigrant Workers Cleaning and Caring in the Shadows of Affluence*. Berkeley: University of California Press.

Hondagneu-Sotelo, Pierette, and Ernestine Avila. 1997. "'I'm here, but I'm there': The meanings of Latina transnational motherhood." *Gender & Society* 11(5):548–571.

Horton, Sarah. 2004. "Different subjects: The health care system's participation in the differential construction of the cultural citizenship of Cuban refugees and Mexican immigrants." *Medical Anthropology Quarterly* 18(4):472–489.

Howes-Mischel, Rebecca. 2010. "Pragmatic logics and embodied mothers: Productions of transnational bodies through modernist narratives of prenatal health." Paper presented at the American Association of Anthropology annual meeting, New Orleans, Louisiana, November 21.

———. Forthcoming. "Local contours of reproductive risk and responsibility in rural Oaxaca." In *The Development of a Discourse Surrounding Reproductive Risk*, edited by Aminata Maraesa and Lauren Fordyce. Nashville, TN: Vanderbilt University Press.

Hunt, L. M., S. Schneider, and B. Comer. 2004. "Should 'acculturation' be a variable in health research? A critical review of research on US Hispanics." *Social Science & Medicine* 59:973–986.

Islas, María. 2010. "Projectivity and transnationalism: Practices of foresight in a migrant community." Paper presented at conference Transnational Citizenship across the Americas, Rutgers University, New Brunswick, New Jersey, March 25.

Ivry, Tsipy. 2010. *Embodying Culture: Pregnancy in Japan and Israel*. New Brunswick, NJ: Rutgers University Press.

Jacoby, Tamar. 2007. "Amnesty's one thing, a solution's another." *Los Angeles Times*, May 10. http://articles.latimes.com/2007/may/10/opinion/oe-jacoby10.

Johnson-Hanks, Jennifer. 2002. "On the Modernity of Traditional Contraception: Time and the Social Context of Fertility." *Population and Development Review* 28: 229–249.

Jones, Ricardo Herbert. 2009. "Teamwork: An obstetrician, a midwife, and a doula in Brazil." In *Birth Models That Work*, edited by Robbie Davis-Floyd, Lesley Barclay, Betty-Anne Daviss, and Jan Tritten, 271–304. Berkeley: University of California Press.

Jordan, Brigitte. 1992. *Technology and Social Interaction: Notes on the Achievement of Authoritative Knowledge.* IRL Technical Report IRL92–0027. Palo Alto, CA: Institute for Research on Learning.

———. 1993. *Birth in Four Cultures.* 4th ed. Prospect Heights, IL: Waveland Press.

———. 1997. "Authoritative knowledge and its construction." In *Childbirth and Authoritative Knowledge,* edited by Robbie Davis-Floyd and Carolyn Sargent, 55–79. Berkeley: University of California Press.

Karpati, A., X. Lu, F. Mostashari, L. Thorpe, and T. R. Frieden. 2003. *The Health of Hunts Point and Mott Haven.* New York: Community Health Profiles.

Kimmel, Tina. 2002. "How the stats really stack up: Cosleeping is twice as safe." *Mothering Magazine* 114, September/October.

Kingsolver, Barbara. 2010. *The Lacuna.* New York: HarperCollins.

Kleinman, Arthur. 1995. *Writing at the Margin: Discourse between Anthropology and Medicine.* Berkeley: University of California Press.

Knight, Al. 2005. "Change U.S. law on anchor babies." *Denver Post,* June 22.

Landale, N. S., R. S. Oropesa, and B. K. Gorman. 1999. "Immigration and infant health: Birth outcomes of immigrant and native-born women." In *Children of Immigrants: Health, Adjustment, and Public Assistance,* edited by D. J. Hernandez, 244–285. Washington, DC: National Academy Press.

———. 2000. "Migration and infant death: Assimilation or selective migration among Puerto Ricans." *American Sociological Review* 65(6):888–909.

Lane, Brenda. 2009. "Epidural rates in the US and around the world." http://childbirth-labour-delivery.suite101.com/article.cfm/epidural_for_labor.

Langer, Ana, and Bernardo Hernández. 2002. "Importancia de los sistemas de referencia en la prevención de la mortalidad materna." *Boletín de Evaluación de Tecnologías para la Salud* (2), April.

Layne, Linda L. 1996. "How's the baby doing? Struggling with narratives of progress in a neonatal intensive care unit." *Medical Anthropology Quarterly* 10(4):624–656.

Lee, Alison Elizabeth. 2008. "'Para salir adelante': The emergence and acceleration of international migration in new sending areas of Puebla, Mexico." *Journal of Latin American and Caribbean Anthropology* 13(1):48–78.

Liu, Kai-Li, and Fabienne Laraque. 2006. "Higher mortality rate among infants of US-born mothers compared to foreign-born mothers in New York City." *Journal of Immigrant and Minority Health* 8(3):281–289.

Magaña, Aizita, and Noreen Clark. 1995. "Examining a paradox: Does religiosity contribute to positive birth outcomes in Mexican American populations?" *Health Education Quarterly* 22(1):96–109.

Maldonado, Andrea. 2010a. *A Members' Only Community: Re-making the Middle Class in Mexico City.* Saarbrücken, Germany: Lambert Academic Publishing.

———. 2010b. "Culture: The new drug of choice in México City." PhD diss. research proposal, Department of Anthropology, Brown University.

Maraesa, Aminata. 2003. *Woman to Woman: Doula Assisted Childbirth.* Film distributed by Documentary Education Resources.

Maraesa, Aminata, and Lauren Fordyce, eds. Forthcoming. *The Development of a Discourse Surrounding Reproductive Risk.* Nashville, TN: Vanderbilt University Press.

Marcelli, Enrico A., and Wayne A. Cornelius. 2001. "The changing profile of Mexican migrants to the United States: New evidence from California and México." *Latin American Research Review* 36(3):105–131.

March of Dimes. 2010. "Low birth weight." *Quick Reference Fact Sheet.* http://www
.marchofdimes.com/professionals/14332_1153.asp#head2.

Marcus, George. 1995. "Ethnography in/of the world system: The emergence of multisited ethnography." *Annual Review of Anthropology* 24:95–117.

Marroni, María Da Gloria. 2003. "The culture of migratory networks: Connecting New
York and Puebla." In *Immigrants and Schooling: Mexicans in New York,* edited by
Regina Cortina and Mónica Gendreau, 125–142. Staten Island, NY: Center for
Migration Studies.

Martin, Emily. 1992. *The Woman in the Body.* 2nd ed. Boston: Beacon Press.

———. 1994. *Flexible Bodies: The Role of Immunity in American Culture from the Days
of Polio to the Age of AIDS.* Boston: Beacon Press.

———. 1996. "Disembodying women: Perspectives on pregnancy and the unborn."
Medical Anthropology Quarterly 10(2):307–309.

Martin, Gary. 2010. "Smith to push enforcement of immigration laws." *My San Antonio
(Express-News),* November 4.

Martin, Joann. 1990. "Motherhood and power: The production of a women's culture of
politics in a Mexican community." *American Ethnologist* 17(3):470–490.

Martin, Joyce A., Brady E. Hamilton, Paul D. Sutton, Stephanie J. Ventura, Fay Menacker,
Sharon Kirmeyer, and T. J. Mathews. 2009. "Births: Final data for 2006." *National
Vital Statistics Report* 57(7).

Martin, Joyce A., and Fay Menacker. 2007. "Expanded health data from the new birth
certificate, 2004." *National Vital Statistics Reports* 55(12):1–23. http://www.cdc.gov/
nchs/data/nvsr/nvsr55/nvsr55_12.pdf.

Marx, Karl. (1852) 2008. *The 18th Brumaire of Louis Bonaparte.* Rockville, MD: Wildside
Press.

Masley, Kate Elizabeth. 2007. "Living the 'Latina paradox': An ethnography of pregnant
and postpartum Mexican immigrants in northeast Ohio." PhD diss., Case Western
Reserve University.

Massey, Douglas S. 1986. "The settlement process among Mexican migrants to the United
States." *American Sociological Review* 51(5):670–684.

Massey, Douglas S., and R. Magaly Sánchez. 2010. *Brokered Boundaries: Creating
Immigrant Identity in Anti-Immigrant Times.* New York: Russell Sage Foundation.

McCarthy, William, Yvonne Flores, Hong Zheng, and Thomas Hanson. 2005. "Immigrant
generational status and ethnic differences in health." *American Journal of Public
Health* 95(9):1494.

McKenna, James J. 2002. "Breastfeeding and bedsharing still useful (and important) after
all these years." *Mothering Magazine* 114, September/October.

Milanich, Nara. 2009. *Children of Fate: Childhood, Class, and the State in Chile,
1850–1930.* Durham, NC: Duke University Press.

Morenoff, Jeffrey David. 2000. "Unraveling paradoxes of public health: Neighborhood
environments and racial/ethnic differences in birth outcomes." PhD diss., University
of Chicago.

Mulvaney-Day, Norah, Margarita Alegría, and William Sribney. 2007. "Social cohesion,
social support, and health among Latinos in the United States." *Social Science &
Medicine* 64:477–495.

Napolitano, Valentina. 2002. *Migration, Mujercitas, and Medicine Men: Living in Urban
México.* Berkeley: University of California Press.

Navarro, Carlos. 2003. "Facing our current challenges." Presentation at a conference at
City College, New York, May 31.

Nelkin, Dorothy. 2003. *Risk, Culture, and Health Inequality: Shifting Perceptions of Danger and Blame*, edited by Barbara Harthorn and Laury Oaks. New York: Praeger.

New York City Department of Health and Mental Hygiene. 2008. *Summary of Vital Statistics 2000–2007*. Accessed August 1, 2008. http://www.nyc.gov/html/doh/html/vs/vs.shtml.

New York State Department of Health. 2010. *2010 PCAP Services Description*. http://www.health.state.ny.us/nysdoh/perinatal/en/servicedescription.htm/.

Newton, Lina. 2008. *Illegal, Alien or Immigrant? The Politics of Immigration Reform*. New York: New York University Press.

Oboler, Suzanne. 2006. "Introduction: Redefining citizenship as lived experience." In *Latinos and Citizenship: The Dilemma of Belonging*, edited by Suzanne Oboler, 1–30. New York: Palgrave Macmillan.

Office of the President of the United States. 2005. *Economic Report of the President*. Washington, DC: U.S. Government Printing Office.

Ong, Aihwa. 1996. "Cultural citizenship as subject-making: Immigrants negotiate racial and cultural boundaries in the United States." *Current Anthropology* 37(5):737–762.

———. 2006. *Neoliberalism as Exception: Mutations in Citizenship and Sovereignty*. Durham, NC: Duke University Press.

Organización de Médicos Indígenas de la Mixteca. 2009. *Organización de Médicos Indígenas de la Mixteca*. Accessed December 15, 2009.http://www.cdi.gob.mx/participacion/omima/situacion.htm.

Pallares, Amalia. 2009. "Impossible activism? Representations of the family in the immigrant rights movement in Chicago." Paper presented at the Undocumented Hispanic Migration conference, Connecticut College, New London, Connecticut, October 16.

———. 2010. "Families untied." Personal communication.

Palloni, Alberto, and Elizabeth Arias. 2004. "Paradox lost: Explaining the Hispanic adult mortality advantage." *Demography* 41(3):385–415.

Palloni, Alberto, and Jeffrey D. Morenoff. 2001. "Interpreting the paradoxical in the Hispanic paradox: Demographic and epidemiologic approaches." *Annals of the New York Academy of Sciences* 954:140–174.

Parker, Jennifer. 1994. "Ethnic differences in midwife-attended U.S. births." *American Journal of Public Health* 84(7):1139–1141.

Parker, Kunal. 2001. "State, citizenship, and territory: The legal construction of immigrants in antebellum Massachusetts." *Law and History Review* 19(3):583–643.

Parrado, Emilio, and Jorge Valencia. 2010. "How high is Mexican/Hispanic fertility in the U.S.?" Working paper, June 22. http://repository.upenn.edu/psc_working_papers/18/.

Passel, Jeffrey. 2005. "Unauthorized migrants: Numbers and characteristics." Pew Hispanic Center. June 14. http://www.pewtrusts.org/uploadedFiles/wwwpewtrustsorg/News/Press_Releases/Hispanics_in_America/PHC_immigrants_0605.pdf.

Passel, Jeffrey, and D'Vera Cohn. 2009. "A portrait of unauthorized immigrants in the United States." Pew Hispanic Center. April 14. http://pewhispanic.org/files/reports/107.pdf.

Pauli, Julia. 2008. "A house of one's own: Gender, migration, and residence in rural México." *American Ethnologist* 35(1):171–187.

Pease Chock, Phyllis. 1996. "No new women: Gender, 'alien,' and 'citizen' in the congressional debate on immigration." *PoLAR* 19(1):1–10.

Pérez Loredo Díaz, Luz. 1991. "Apuntes sobre las parteras y el arte de los partos durante el virreinato." *Revista de Enfermería*, Instituto Mexicano del Seguro Social (México) 4(1):53–55.

Petchesky, Rosalind. 1998. "Introduction." In *Negotiating Reproductive Rights*, edited by Rosalind Petchesky and Karen Judd, 1–30. New York: Palgrave.

Piven, Frances Fox, and Richard Cloward. 1971. *Regulating the Poor: The Functions of Public Welfare*. New York: Random House.

Portes, Alejandro, and Rubén G. Rumbaut. 2001. *Legacies: The Story of the Immigrant Second Generation*. Berkeley: University of California Press.

Portes, Alejandro, and Min Zhou. 1993. "The new second generation: Segmented assimilation and its variants." *Annals of the American Academy of Political and Social Science* 530 (November):74–96.

President of the Republic of Mexico. 2009. "International Women's Day." Press release. May 28. http://www.presidencia.gob.mx/en/press/?contenido=45307.

Pritchard, Justin. 2004. "A Mexican worker dies each day, A. P. finds." *Newsday,* March 14.

Putnam, Robert D. 1993. "The prosperous community: Social capital and economic growth." *Current* 356:4–6.

Rabinow, Paul. 1992. "Artificiality and enlightenment: From sociobiology to biosociality." In *Incorporations,* edited by Jonathan Crary and Sanford Kwinter, 234–251. New York: Zone Books.

Raison, Eva Blom. 2007. "Pidiendo la palabra: Immigrant narratives and Spanish literacy in New York City." Master's thesis, New York University.

Ramírez Carillo, Cristina. 2001. "Evolución del cuidado materno infantil." *Revista de Enfermería*, Instituto Mexicano del Seguro Social (México) 9(1):1–4.

Rapp, Rayna. 2000. *Testing Women, Testing the Fetus: The Social Impact of Amniocentesis in America*. New York: Routledge.

Rivera Batiz, Francisco. 2002. *The Socioeconomic Status of Hispanic New Yorkers: Current Trends and Future Prospects*. Pew Hispanic Center Study: A Project of the Pew Charitable Trusts and USC Annenberg School for Communication. http://eric .ed.gov:80/PDFS/ED465825.pdf.

Rivera Sánchez, Liliana. 2002. Personal communication.

Roberts, Sam. 2006. "The 300 millionth American, don't ask who." *New York Times,* October 18. http://www.nytimes.com/2006/10/18/us/18population.html.

Rodriguez, Gregory. 2008. *Bastards, Mongrels, Orphans, and Vagabonds: Mexican Immigration and the Future of Race in America*. New York: Vintage Books.

Root, Robin, and Carole H. Browner. 2001. "Practices of the pregnant self: Compliance with and resistance to prenatal norms." *Culture, Medicine and Psychiatry* 25:195–223.

Rose, Nikolas, and Carlos Novas. 2005. "Biological citizenship." In *Global Assemblages: Technology, Politics, and Ethics as Anthropological Problems*, edited by Aihwa Ong and Stephen Collier, 439–463. Oxford: Blackwell.

Rothenberg, S. J., M. Manalo, and J. Jiang. 1999. "Maternal blood leads level during pregnancy in South Central Los Angeles." *Archives of Environmental Health* 54:151–157.

Ruíz-Navarro, Patricia. 2009. *Fertility Rates among Mexicans in Traditional and New States of Settlement 2006*. Report 27, Center for Latin American, Caribbean and Latino Studies, Graduate Center of the City University of New York. November.

Rumbaut, R. G., and J. R. Weeks. 1996. "Unraveling a public health enigma: Why do immigrants experience superior peri-natal health outcomes?" *Research in the Sociology of Health Care* 13(B):337–391.

Sahagún, Bernardino de. (1561–1582) 1950. *Florentine Codex: General History of the Things of New Spain 1561–82*. Santa Fe, NM: School of American Research and the University of Utah.

Santiago-Irizarry, Vilma. 1996. "Culture as cure." *Cultural Anthropology* 11(1):3–24.

Santora, Marc. 2006. "East meets west, adding pounds and peril." *New York Times*, January 12.

Sargent, Carolyn, and Grace Bascope. 1996. "Ways of knowing about birth in three cultures." *Medical Anthropology Quarterly* 10(2):213–236.

Sargent, Carolyn, and Nancy Stark. 1989. "Childbirth education and childbirth models: Parental perspectives on control, anesthesia, and technological intervention in the birth process." *Medical Anthropology Quarterly* 3(1):36–51.

Schirmer, Jennifer. 1993. "The seeking of truth and the gendering of consciousness: The COMADRES of El Salvador and the CONAVIGUA widows of Guatemala." In *Viva: Women and Popular Protest in Latin America,* edited by Sarah A. Radcliffe and Sallie Westwood, 30–64. London: Routledge.

Schwartz, Steven, and Wenhui Li. 2002. *Summary of Vital Statistics 2001.* New York: City of New York.

———. 2003. *Summary of Vital Statistics 2002.* New York: City of New York.

———. 2004. *Summary of Vital Statistics 2003.* New York: City of New York.

Schwartz, Steven, Regina Zimmerman, and Wenhui Li. 2005. *Summary of Vital Statistics 2004.* New York: City of New York.

———. 2006. *Summary of Vital Statistics 2005.* New York: City of New York.

Scott, Joan. 1992. "Experience." In *Feminists Theorize the Political,* edited by Judith Butler and J. W. Scott, 22–40. London: Routledge.

Scribner, Richard. 1996. "Paradox as paradigm: The health outcomes of Mexican Americans." *American Journal of Public Health* 86(3):303–305.

Scribner, Richard, and J. H. Dwyer. 1989. "Acculturation and low birthweight among Latinos in the Hispanic HANES." *American Journal of Public Health* 79(9):1263–1267.

Secretaría de la Salud. 2002. *Arranque Parejo en la Vida.* http://www.salud.gob.mx/docprog/estrategia_2/arranque_parejo_vida.pdf.

Sesia, Paola. 1996. "Women come here on their own when they need to: Prenatal care, authoritative knowledge, and maternal health in Oaxaca." *Medical Anthropology Quarterly* 10(2):121–141.

Shai, D., and I. Rosenwaike. 1987. "Mortality among Hispanics in metropolitan Chicago: An examination based on vital statistics data." *Journal of Chronic Disease* 40:445–451.

Sherraden, Margaret, and Rossana Barrera. 1996. "Maternal support and cultural influences among Mexican immigrant mothers." *Families in Society* 77(5):298–313.

Shierholz, Heidi. 2010. "Immigration and wages—Methodological advancements confirm modest gains for native workers." Economic Policy Institute, February 4. http://www.epi.org/publications/entry/bp255/.

Sider, Gerald. 2003. *Between History and Tomorrow: Making and Breaking Everyday Life in Rural Newfoundland.* Toronto: Broadview Press.

Simpson, Ellen, Timothy Gowron, Dennis Mull, and Ann P. Walker. 1994. "A Spanish-language prenatal family health evaluation questionnaire: Construction and pilot implementation." *Journal of Genetic Counseling* 3:39–62.

Simpson, Ellen, J. Dennis Mull, Erin Longley, and Joan East. 2000. "Pica during pregnancy in low-income women born in México." *Western Journal of Medicine* 173(1):20–24.

Singh, G. K., and M. Siahpush. 2001. "All-cause and cause-specific mortality of immigrants and native born in the United States." *American Journal of Public Health* 91(3):392–400.

Siulc, Nina. 2003. "The right to be respected: The politics of health care among Mexican immigrants in New York City." Paper presented at the American Anthropological Association Annual Meetings, Chicago, November 21.

Smith, Robert C. 2005. *Mexicans in New York*. Berkeley: University of California Press.

Smith-Oka, Vania. 2009. "Unintended consequences: Exploring the tensions between development programs and indigenous women in México in the context of reproductive health." *Social Science and Medicine* 68:2069–2077.

———. Forthcoming. "Risking body and child: Biomedical and local perceptions of pregnancy and birth in Mexico." In *The Development of a Discourse Surrounding Reproductive Risk*, edited by Aminata Maraesa and Lauren Fordyce. Nashville, TN: Vanderbilt University Press.

So, Jimmy. 2010. "Kyl: Illegal Aliens' Kids Shouldn't Be Citizens." CBS News, August 1. http://www.cbsnews.com/stories/2010/08/01/ftn/main6733905.shtml.

Sointu, Eeva. 2006. "The search for wellbeing in alternative and complementary health practices." *Sociology of Health & Illness* 28(3):330–349.

Solís, Jocelyn, Genoveva García, and Silvana Bonil. 2002. "Mexican women's community response to domestic violence: A sociocultural analysis of migration, gender and violence." Paper presented at the Hominis Intercontinental Convention, Havana, Cuba, November 4–8.

Somerville, Will, and Madeleine Sumption. 2009. "Immigration and the labour market: Theory, evidence, and policy." Equality and Human Rights Commission. http://www.migrationpolicy.org/pubs/Immigration-and-the-Labour-Market.pdf.

Sorlie, P. D., E. Backlund, N. J. Johnson, and E. Rogot. 1993. "Mortality by Hispanic status in the United States." *Journal of the American Medical Association* 270:2464–2468.

Steinweg, Carrie. 2010. "American College of Obstetricians and Gynecologists relaxes VBAC guidelines." *Chicago Examiner*, July 24. http://www.examiner.com/family-in-chicago/american-college-of-obstetricians-and-gynecologists-relaxes-vbac-guidelines.

Stephen, Lynn. 1991. *Zapotec Women*. Austin: University of Texas Press.

Sterling, Terry Greene. 2010. "FAIR-y tales." *Village Voice*, December 1. http://www.villagevoice.com/2010–12–01/news/fairy-y-tales/.

Strong, Thomas. 2000. *Expecting Trouble: What Expectant Parents Should Know about Prenatal Care in America*. New York: New York University Press.

Suárez-Orozco, Marcelo. 2009. Plenary lecture, presented at the Undocumented Hispanic Migration conference, Connecticut College, New London, Connecticut, October 17.

Susser, Merwyn. 1973. *Causal Thinking in the Social Sciences: Concepts and Strategies of Epidemiology*. New York: Oxford University Press.

Szreter, Simon. 1993. "The idea of demographic transition and the study of fertility change: A critical intellectual history." *Population and Development Review* 19(4):659–701.

Taningco, María Teresa V. 2007. *Revisiting the Latino Health Paradox*. Policy Brief. Tomás Rivera Policy Institute, Los Angeles. August.

Thompson, Ginger. 2006. "Some in México see border wall as opportunity." *New York Times*, May 25.

Thorpe, Lorna, Diana Berger, Jennifer A. Ellis, Vani R. Bettegowda, Gina Brown, Thomas Matte, Mary Bassett, and Thomas R. Frieden. 2005. "Trends and racial/ethnic disparities in gestational diabetes among pregnant women in New York City." *American Journal of Public Health* 95(9):1536–1538.

Tyson, Peter. 2004. *History of Quarantine*. August. http://www.pbs.org/wgbh/nova/typhoid/quarantine.html.

U.S. Census Bureau. 2005. *American Community Survey*. Washington, DC.

———.2006. *American Community Survey*. Washington, DC.

————.2007. *American Community Survey*. Washington, DC.

————.2008. *American Community Survey*. Washington, DC.

————. 2010. *Census 2010*. http://2010.census.gov/2010census/.

U.S. Census Monitoring Board. 2001. *Final Report to Congress*. http://govinfo.library .unt.edu/cmb/cmbp/reports/final_report/fin_sec5_effect.pdf.

U.S. Department of Agriculture. 2010. *WIC Food Packages*. http://www.fns.usda.gov/ wic/benefitsandservices/foodpkg.htm.

United Nations. 2000. "2000 Millennium Development Goals." http://www.un.org/ millenniumgoals/maternal.shtml.

Unnatural Causes. 2007. Documentary film. California News Reel.

Urban Baby. 2010. Postings such as "Two weeks pregnant with #2 and craving a glass of wine." http://www.urbanbaby.com/talk/posts/51978078.

Valenzuela, Angela. 1999. *Subtractive Schooling: U.S.-Mexican Youth and the Politics of Caring*. Albany: State University of New York Press.

van der Geest, Sjaak, and Kaja Finkler. 2004. "Hospital ethnography: Introduction." *Social Science & Medicine* 59(10):1995–2001.

Van Teijlingen, Edwin R., George W. Lowis, Peter McCaffery, and Maureen Porter. 2004. *Midwifery and the Medicalization of Childbirth: Comparative Perspectives*. Hauppauge, NY: Nova Science.

Vanderpool, Tim. 2008. "Price of admission: Along the border, sexual assault has become routine." *Tucson Weekly*, June 5.

Vega, William A., and Hortensia Amaro. 1994. "Latino outlook: Good health, uncertain prognosis." *Annual Review of Public Health* 15:39–67.

Vega, William A., M. A. Rodríguez, and E. Gruskin. 2009. "Health disparities in the Latino population." *Epidemiological Review* 31(1):99–112.

Velasco, Vitelio. 2002. "La mortalidad materna en el IMSS: Los aspectos médicos de un problema multifactorial." *Boletín de Evaluación de Tecnologías para la Salud* (2), April.

Viladrich, Anahí. 2003. "Social careers, social capital, and immigrants' access barriers to health care: The case of the Argentine minority in New York City." PhD diss., Columbia University.

————. 2009. "From entitlement to undeservedness: The legacy of welfare reform." Paper presented at the Undocumented Hispanic Migration conference, Connecticut College, New London, Connecticut, October 17.

Viruell-Fuentes, Edna A. 2006. "A Critical Analysis of the Latino Health Paradox through the Narratives of Mexican Immigrant Women." Paper presented at the 26th International Congress of the Latin American Studies Association, San Juan, Puerto Rico, March 18.

Viruell-Fuentes, Edna A., and A. J. Schulz. 2009. "Toward a dynamic conceptualization of social ties and context: Implications for understanding immigrant and Latino health." *American Journal of Public Health* 99(12):2167–2175.

Wailoo, Keith, Julie Livingston, and Peter Guarnaccia. 2006. "Introduction: Chronicles of an accidental death." In *A Death Retold: Jesica Santillán, the Bungled Transplant, and Paradoxes of Medical Citizenship*, edited by Keith Wailoo, Julie Livingston, and Peter Gaurnaccia, 1–16. Chapel Hill: University of North Carolina Press.

Wallace, Rodrick, and Deborah Wallace. 1998. *A Plague on Your Houses: How New York Was Burned Down and National Public Health Crumbled*. London, New York: Verso.

Werbner, Pnina. 1999. "Political motherhood and the feminisation of citizenship: Women's activisms and the transformation of the public sphere." In *Women, Citizenship, and*

Difference, edited by Nira Yuval-Davis and Pnina Werbner, 221–245. London: Zed Books.

Williams, Ronald, Nancy Binkin, and Elizabeth Clingman. 1986. "Pregnancy outcomes among Spanish-surname women in California." *American Journal of Public Health* 76:387–391.

Wilson, Ellen K. 2008. "Acculturation and changes in the likelihood of pregnancy and feelings about pregnancy among women of Mexican origin." *Women & Health* 47(1):45–64.

World Bank. 2008. "The South teaches the North how to break the cycle of poverty." February 11. http://web.worldbank.org/WBSITE/EXTERNAL/NEWS/0,,contentMDK: 21642718~pagePK:64257043~piPK:437376~theSitePK:4607,00.html.

———. 2010. *World Bank Development Indicators.* http://data.worldbank.org/data-catalog/world-development-indicators?cid=GPD_WDI.

Yuval-Davis, Nira, and Pnina Werbner. 1999. "Introduction." In *Women, Citizenship, and Difference,* edited by Nira Yuval-Davis and Pnina Werbner, 1–38. London: Zed Books.

Index

Note: Page references in *italics* refer to photographs.

About the Author

Alyshia Gálvez (Ph.D. Anthropology, New York University, 2004) is an assistant professor of Latin American and Puerto Rican Studies at Lehman College, City University of New York. This is her second single-authored book. Her first, *Guadalupe in New York: Devotion and the Struggle for Citizenship Rights among Mexicans in New York* (New York University Press, 2009), examines the efforts of Mexican immigrants to achieve the rights of citizenship through activism in devotional organizations dedicated to the Virgin of Guadalupe. In addition, she edited the book *Performing Religion in the Americas* and the special issue of the journal *e-misférica* titled "Traveling Virgins/Virgenes Viajeras."

Available titles in the Critical Issues in Health and Medicine series:

Heather Munro Prescott, *The Morning After: A History of Emergency Contraception in the United States*

David G. Schuster, *Neurasthenic Nation: America's Search for Health, Happiness, and Comfort, 1869–1920*

Karen Seccombe and Kim A. Hoffman, *Just Don't Get Sick: Access to Health Care in the Aftermath of Welfare Reform*

Leo B. Slater, *War and Disease: Biomedical Research on Malaria in the Twentieth Century*

Matthew Smith, *An Alternative History of Hyperactivity: Food Additives and the Feingold Diet*

Rosemary A. Stevens, Charles E. Rosenberg, and Lawton R. Burns, eds., *History and Health Policy in the United States: Putting the Past Back In*

Barbra Mann Wall, *American Catholic Hospitals: A Century of Changing Markets and Missions*

CPSIA information can be obtained at www.ICGtesting.com
Printed in the USA
270081BV00003B/3/P